# Lecture Notes in Information Systems and Organisation

## Volume 17

More information about this series at http://www.springer.com/series/11237

Doug Vogel · Xitong Guo · Henry Linger
Chris Barry · Michael Lang
Christoph Schneider
Editors

# Transforming Healthcare Through Information Systems

Proceedings of the 24th International
Conference on Information Systems
Development

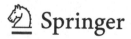 Springer

*Editors*
Doug Vogel
Harbin Institute of Technology
Harbin
China

Xitong Guo
Harbin Institute of Technology
Harbin
China

Henry Linger
Caulfield School of Information Technology
Monash University
Caulfield East, VIC
Australia

Chris Barry
J.E. Cairnes School of Business &
    Economics
National University of Ireland
Galway
Ireland

Michael Lang
J.E. Cairnes School of Business &
    Economics
National University of Ireland
Galway
Ireland

Christoph Schneider
City University of Hong Kong
Kowloon
Hong Kong

ISSN 2195-4968            ·            ISSN 2195-4976   (electronic)
Lecture Notes in Information Systems and Organisation
ISBN 978-3-319-30132-7        ISBN 978-3-319-30133-4   (eBook)
DOI 10.1007/978-3-319-30133-4

Library of Congress Control Number: 2016932860

Printed on acid-free paper

This Springer imprint is published by Springer Nature
The registered company is Springer International Publishing AG Switzerland

# Preface

The *International Conference on Information Systems Development* (ISD) is an academic conference where researchers and practitioners share their knowledge and expertise in the field of information systems development. As an Affiliated Conference of the Association for Information Systems (AIS), the ISD conference complements the international network of general IS conferences (ICIS, ECIS, AMCIS, PACIS, ACIS). The ISD conference continues the tradition started with the first Polish-Scandinavian Seminar on Current Trends in Information Systems Development Methodologies, held in Gdansk, Poland in 1988. This seminar has evolved into the International Conference on Information Systems Development.

During its history, the conference has focused on different aspects, ranging from methodological, infrastructural, or educational challenges in the ISD field to bridging the gaps between industry, academia, and society. The development of information systems has paralleled technological developments and the deployment of those technologies in all areas of society, including government, industry, community, and in the home. ISD has always promoted a close interaction between theory and practice that has set an agenda focused on the integration of people, processes, and technology within a specific context.

This publication is a selection of papers from ISD2015, the 24th ISD conference hosted by the eHealth Research Institute, School of Management, Harbin Institute of Technology and held in Harbin, China during August 25–27, 2015. All accepted papers for ISD2015 have been published in the AIS eLibrary at http://aisel.aisnet.org/isd2014/proceedings2015. This volume contains extended versions of the best papers, as selected by the ISD2015 Program Chairs.

The theme of the conference was *Transforming Healthcare through Information Systems*. Healthcare as we know it is increasingly unaffordable and incapable of dealing with emerging population dynamics. The combination of increased life expectancy coupled with high incidence of chronic and lifestyle diseases creates an overwhelming demand on healthcare facilities and professionals. No country in the world can continue to provide broad-based quality healthcare under these circumstances without new thinking. The issues are many and the stakeholder list is long, leading to the societal challenges we now face.

Information systems play an important role in healthcare transformation to meet the current and future needs. As healthcare expands to address wellness as well as treatment in a more patient-centric context, aspects of content and process as well as technology all enter into Information System Development considerations. Opportunities are especially salient given the current prevalence of emergent technologies for a broad range of uses and a historical lack of attention to the problem of integration within the health system.

New healthcare thinking also requires sustained behavioral change that cannot be mandated. As such, information systems need to be both technologically robust and also appealing to broad segments of the population. Implementation needs to address a wide range of issues so that systems are used and are useful in terms of long-term benefits and positive impacts on healthcare systems.

The ISD2015 conference tracks focused on:

- IS Impact on Healthcare Organizations and Society
- ISD Education
- Sensor-Based Systems Development
- Mobile Systems and Applications
- Model-Driven Development and Concepts
- Security and Privacy Considerations
- General Concepts e.g., Managing IS Development, ISD Methodologies, Project Management, Innovation in ISD, Legal/Ethical Issues, and Other Topics.

The ISD2015 conference focused on these and associated topics in order to promote research into methodological issues and ways in which information systems designers are transforming healthcare. We believe that the papers assembled in this publication are an important contribution in this regard.

Doug Vogel
Xitong Guo
Henry Linger
Chris Barry
Michael Lang
Christoph Schneider

# Conference Organization

## Conference Chair

Qiang Ye

## Program Chairs

Doug Vogel
Xitong Guo

## Organizing Committee Chairs

Xiaofeng Ju
Hua Lan

## International Steering Committee

Chris Barry
Michael Lang
Henry Linger
Christoph Schneider

## Track Chairs

### IS Impact on Healthcare Organizations and Society
Joe Valacich
Xunhua Guo
Yongqiang Sun

**ISD for Healthcare Education**

Mark Freeman
Kanliang Wang
ZeyuPeng

**Sensor-Based Systems Development**

Dongsong Zhang
Jacky Zhang

**Mobile Systems and Applications**

Christer Carlsson
Cheng Zhang

**Model-Driven Development and Concepts**

William Wei
Sheng Zhang
Tianshi Wu

**Security and Privacy Considerations**

Paul Lowry
Chul Ho Lee

**General Concepts (Including ISD Methodologies, Project Management, and Other Topics)**

Jiye Mao
Nilmini Wickramasinghe
Huaiqing Wang
Kaiquan Xu

# Reviewers

Somayeh Aghanavesi
Ahmad Alaiad
Tong Che
Hui Chen
Jin Chen
Wen Yong Chua
Yuanyuan Dang
Carmelo Del Valle
Xiaofeng Du
Maria Jose Escalona
Michael Frutiger
Yang Gao
Cong Geng
Huijing Guo
Shanshan Guo
Xitong Guo

Alberto Gutierrez-Escolar
Haibo Hu
Liqiang Huang
Lei Jing
Lele Kang
Gunes Koru
Ming Lei
Jia Li
Yan Li
Fei Liu
Guannan Liu
Luning Liu
Xiaoxiao Liu
Xuan Liu
Zhiyong Liu
Marcos López-Sanz
Fanbo Meng
Xiangli Meng
Yao Meng
Peng Ouyang
Malgorzata Pankowska
Jiajun Pei
German Retana
Zhen Shao
Xiao-Liang Shen
Rax Chun Lung Suen
Liuan Wang
Hong Wu
Hao Xia
Gang Xue
Xiangda Yan
Hualong Yang
Zi Yang
Hua Yuan
Huiru Yuan
Shaozhong Zhang
Sheng Zhang
Xiaofei Zhang
Yuan Zhang
Xiaoyun Zhao
Zhongyun Zhou

# Contents

# A Method for Systematic Adaptation and Synchronization of Healthcare Processes

Álvaro E. Prieto, Adolfo Lozano-Tello,
Roberto Rodríguez-Echeverría and Fernando Sánchez-Figueroa

**Abstract** International organizations, as the World Health Organization (WHO), are constantly defining new healthcare protocols and procedures, as well as modifying previously adopted ones. As a result, most health institutions have to adapt continuously their workflows and information systems in order to be aligned with international standards. This problem, called Hierarchical Adaptation Problem, is common in hierarchical domains that use administrative workflows. It also implies establishing the change propagation methods to maintain the consistency among the different levels when the original workflow is changed. To solve this problem, this work introduces the Hierarchical Adaptation Method. A method based on ontologies to define the rules that must be satisfied by a generic workflow to be considered adaptable to different application cases and the rules that must be satisfied by its adapted versions. Moreover, it provides the operations to facilitate both adaptation of workflows and propagation of changes.

**Keywords** Workflows · Ontologies · Hierarchical adaptation · Propagation

A prior version of this paper has been published in the ISD2015 Proceedings (http://aisel.aisnet.org/isd2014/proceedings2015/).

Á.E. Prieto (✉) · A. Lozano-Tello · R. Rodríguez-Echeverría · F. Sánchez-Figueroa
Quercus Software Engineering Group, University of Extremadura,
Cáceres, Spain
e-mail: aeprieto@unex.es

A. Lozano-Tello
e-mail: alozano@unex.es

R. Rodríguez-Echeverría
e-mail: rre@unex.es

F. Sánchez-Figueroa
e-mail: Fernando@unex.es

© Springer International Publishing Switzerland 2016
D. Vogel et al. (eds.), *Transforming Healthcare Through Information Systems*,
Lecture Notes in Information Systems and Organisation 17,
DOI 10.1007/978-3-319-30133-4_1

# 1 Introduction

International organizations, as the World Health Organization (WHO) and national governments are constantly defining or modifying new healthcare protocols and procedures. It produces a significant impact, on one side, on the organizational concerns of a great number of healthcare institutions and centers, and on the other side, on their health information systems that need to be adapted according to these definitions. Most of these healthcare processes can be considered as a special kind of administrative processes.

Administrative processes are a type of business processes widely used in public institutions and large companies. These processes are characterized by being governed by laws, regulations or well-defined action rules that define clearly which activities should be performed, their order, who must perform each activity, how each one must be done and how much time is available for doing them [1, 2].

Workflows are used for automatically managing different types of business processes as administrative processes [3]. Workflows for administrative processes (hereinafter referred to as administrative workflows) have distinctive features that distinguish them from other type of workflows. Those workflows are intended for predictable and repetitive processes. And they must have mechanisms that enable the coordination of the users responsible of each activity, including the notification of deadlines for completing them [4–6]. Normally, these workflows do not have to manage a considerable number of activities, users or data. Problems arise when the organizations need to use them in their different areas and departments, which means that the workflow specification must be adapted to the particular conditions of each area but conforming to the general specification established by the law or regulation that rules the process. This problem is called Hierarchical Adaptation Problem.

The Hierarchical Adaptation Problem (hereinafter referred to as HAP) may appear when an administrative process should be consequently adapted to the specific characteristics of every institution to be applied, but those modifications should not affect the restrictions defined in the original workflow specification. Moreover, HAP implies the necessity of a synchronization strategy between the original workflow and all its different versions, i.e. any change in the original workflow should be properly propagated to every version. This problem implies, on one hand, keeping the consistency of the administrative processes at the different levels of an organization and, on the other hand, if the law or regulation that rules the generic process is changed, establishing the measures that must be taken in order to propagate those changes to the adaptations made in the different areas and departments.

This paper presents an approach to solve this problem called Hierarchical Adaptation Method. This method is based on the specification of administrative workflows by means of ontologies. So, the method establishes the rules that verify the correctness of a workflow specification by means of ontologies, the rules that must satisfy the ontology of a generic workflow to be considered adaptable to different application scenarios and the rules that must satisfy the adaptations of the ontology. Moreover, they provide the set of operations that allow users to make the adaptations correctly and to propagate changes from adaptable workflows to adapted workflows.

As an example to illustrate the stages proposed in the method, the process to define the adaptation framework and to get adapted versions of a real healthcare workflow is presented. This workflow is inspired in the process to apply for inclusion on the Spanish Rare Disease Registry.[1] This is a national level process that each Spanish regional government may adapt to its special circumstances without altering original restrictions.

This paper is structured as follows: Sect. 2 describes the Hierarchical Adaptation Method, Sect. 3 identifies related work, and Sect. 4 presents main conclusions.

## 2 Hierarchical Adaptation Method

A hierarchical workflow adaptation is basically conformed by four interrelated stages:

1. Generic (original) workflow specification. In this first stage, a generic workflow is specified following the process defined by the general regulation. The specification language should provide the engineers with the proper features to specify activities, their order and deadlines, their data and who is in charge of them. The specification language should also allow defining adaptation restrictions over any element of the workflow. The final product of this stage is the specification of the generic workflow managing the administrative process.
2. Specification of adaptation restrictions. In this second stage, engineers should indicate which elements must be always present in any possible version of the original workflow by defining adaptation restrictions. The final result of this stage is the specification of the adaptable workflow.
3. Adaptation. Taking as input the adaptable workflow and taking into account the specific features of the adaptation case (context), the adapted workflow is defined. The final product of this stage is a properly adapted workflow.
4. Propagation. This is an optional stage. It should be carried out when the generic workflow is modified. Then it is mandatory to modify conveniently the adaptable workflow. And then all those changes should be propagated to every adapted workflow. The final products of this stage are the new version of the adaptable workflow and the new versions of every adapted workflow.

The Hierarchical Adaptation Method (hereinafter referred to as HAM) is based on the specification of workflows by means of ontologies. This is due to the several advantages that the use of ontologies can provide to solve the HAP. Firstly, its completeness, flexibility and accuracy for representing workflows, specifying, not

---

[1]https://spainrdr.isciii.es/en/Pages/default.aspx.

only the activities, but also the participants and the data involved together with the characteristics of adaptation of each of these elements in each workflow. Secondly, it allows dividing workflow specifications into two ontologies. One ontology with the relevant data of the domain and the users which can participate in the workflow and another one with the properties of the process and the activities that the process contains, its order, what type of user of the first ontology can perform the activities and what data of the first ontology and what process properties will be managed by every activity. This division will facilitate both the reuse of data and workflows participants from the same domain as the adaptation of workflows to particular cases. Thirdly, the use of ontologies allows a more open notion of adaptation. This is due to the designer of the generic workflow will be who establish the particular adaptation restrictions of each workflow. Lastly, the specification of workflows in ontologies, where each element has a clearly defined purpose, facilitates the development of the set of propagation operations that are necessary to broadcast any change from the generic workflow to its adapted workflows.

On this basis, HAM provides the methods and operations needed to deal with each of the four stages that constitute the HAP. For the first stage, it supplies the ontology *OntoMetaWorkflow* and the method that, using this ontology, allows specifying administrative workflows in two ontologies, called *OntoDD* and *OntoWF*. For the second stage, it defines the set of adaptation restrictions that can be established on a workflow specified in *OntoDD* and *OntoWF* ontologies. Moreover, it provides the rules that must be satisfied establishing these restrictions in order to consider the workflow as an adaptable workflow. The method that allows setting these restrictions in a correct manner is also provided. For the third stage, the Method defines the rules that must satisfy a workflow to be considered a properly adapted workflow of an adaptable workflow. Furthermore, it provides the complete set of hierarchical adaptation operations for specifying correctly an adapted workflow from an adaptable workflow. Lastly, for the fourth stage, it provides the complete set of hierarchical propagation operations. These operations allow that any change affecting the adaptable workflow, over time, can be hierarchically propagated to its adapted workflows.

The following subsections describe how to deal with each of the stages of the Hierarchical Adaptation Problem by means of the concepts and operations of the Hierarchical Adaptation Method.


## 2.1   First Stage: Specification of the Generic Workflow

For the first stage, the approach for representing administrative workflows in ontologies proposed in [7] and restructured in [8] has been updated in the Hierarchical Adaptation Method.

Thus, the specification of the generic workflow is going to be made using the *OntoMetaWorkflow* ontology. This ontology provides the framework for representing administrative workflows defining the common elements of them. Using

*OntoMetaWorkflow*, an ontology engineer must build, in first place, the *OntoDD* ontology. This ontology will contain the relevant data of a particular domain and the users that could participate in the workflows of that domain. Secondly, the ontology engineer will specify the logic of the administrative workflow in an ontology called *OntoWF*. *OntoWF* will contain the particular properties of an administrative workflow together with its activities, the order of execution of said activities, what users, specified in *OntoDD*, can perform the activities and what properties of the workflow specified in *OntoWF* and what domain data specified in *OntoDD* can be shown or modified in an activity.

In order to solve the HAP, *OntoMetaWorkflow* has been extended with a set of elements to specify adaptation restrictions over a concrete workflow. They are used since the second stage and are detailed in the next subsection. The elements of *OntoMetaWorkflow* used in this first stage are the specification elements. These elements serve to specify the activities of the workflow, the users that will perform the activities and the data used in the entire process. These elements together with the way they are used in *OntoDD* and *OntoWF* ontologies are shown in Fig. 1. A detailed explanation of these elements and the method for specifying administrative workflows in ontologies using them is available in [8].

Moreover, in order to deal with the rest of the stages of the Problem, 24 basic modification operations (not shown in this work), has been developed. These operations can be applied on a workflow specified using *OntoMetaWorkflow*

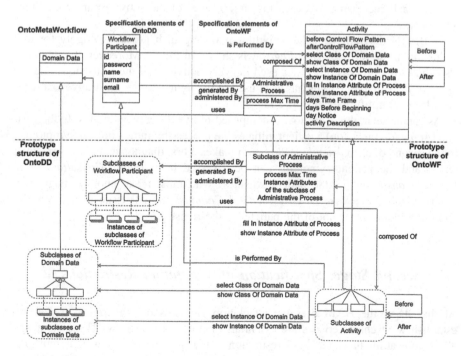

**Fig. 1** Specification elements of OntoMetaWorkflow

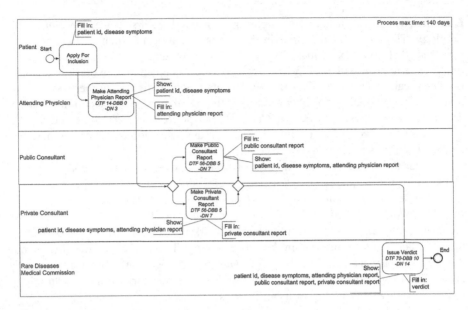

**Fig. 2** Rare Disease Registry inclusion process

keeping the correctness of the workflow. They allow adding and removing different elements and increasing and reducing time frames of the activities and the entire workflow.

A BPMN diagram with the activities of the Spanish process to apply for the inclusion on the *Rare Disease Registry* is shown in Fig. 2. Moreover, the diagram also shows the process properties used in every activity and the restrictions related to the days available. BPMN has been used in the figures of the illustrative example in order to simplify their understanding.

As can be seen, this workflow is composed of five different activities. In the first one (*Apply for Inclusion*) a patient initiates the process by indicating her symptoms. In the second one, an *Attending Physician* makes a first diagnostic report. Next, this report and the patient symptoms can be assessed by a *Public Consultant* or a *Private Consultant* (as the patient whishes) who must make another diagnostic report. Finally, the *Rare Disease Medical Commission* will issue a final verdict about the inclusion or not of the patient on the registry.

## 2.2   Second Stage: Specification of Adaptation Restrictions

At this stage, the HAM uses the adaptation elements of *OntoMetaWorkflow* to establish what characteristics are essentials or not in a workflow. These elements allow indicating the adaptation restrictions of a generic workflow that must be satisfied in any possible adaptation of it. Moreover, the correct use of these elements will ensure that the adapted workflows are valid hierarchical adaptations from the generic workflow.

Three types of adaptation elements have been defined in *OntoMetaWorkflow*: *Mandatory*, Rigid and *Required*.

The first type of elements is used to indicate what activities (with *Mandatory Activities*), participants (with *Mandatory* Participants) and domain data and properties (with *Mandatory Data*) must always be in any possible adaptation of a workflow.

The second type is composed only of Boolean properties that are used within the activities to indicate that some of the relationships between them and the rest of elements cannot be modified in the adapted workflows. So, *Rigid Before* and *Rigid After* will indicate that the activities located immediately before and after of the activity must be always the same. *Rigid Participants* will not allow modifying the participants that can perform the activity. *Rigid Updateable Data* and *Rigid Viewable Data* will indicate that the domain data and the properties that a participant can select, modify or simply read in the activity cannot be changed in the adapted workflows. And, at last, *Rigid Days Time Frame* and *Rigid Days Before Beginning* don't allow modify the time frame and the days before beginning the activity. This means that if an adapted workflow cannot satisfy these restrictions for any activity, it is necessary to remove such activity from the adapted workflow.

The last type is also used within the activities, but in this case it will only indicate minimum requirements and it will not limit the possibility of adding new elements in the adapted workflows. So, in *Required Before* and in *Required After* will be indicated which activities, at least, must be located before and after the activity and, in *Required Participants*, which participants, at least, must be available to perform the activity. In the same way, *Required Updateable Data* and *Required Viewable Data* will indicate which domain data and properties, at least, can select, modify or simply read a participant during the activity. As with the second type of elements, if any activity of the adapted workflow cannot satisfy these restrictions, it is necessary to remove such activity from the adapted workflow.

These elements together with the way they are used in *OntoDD* and *OntoWF* ontologies are shown in Fig. 3.

Using these adaptation elements, at this stage of the HAM is established the formal definition of adaptable workflow. So, an adaptable workflow will be a workflow correctly specified using *OntoMetaWorkflow* and whose values in the adaptations elements satisfy the next restriction: the workflow exclusively composed by the activities, participants, domain data, and process properties indicated in the *Mandatory* elements must be, by itself, a workflow correctly specified using *OntoMetaWorkflow*. This definition implies that it is not possible indicate arbitrary values in the adaptation elements; on the contrary, these values must be coherent. In order to facilitate the correct specification of adaptable workflows, HAM provides a method to correctly specify an adaptable workflow following the next steps:

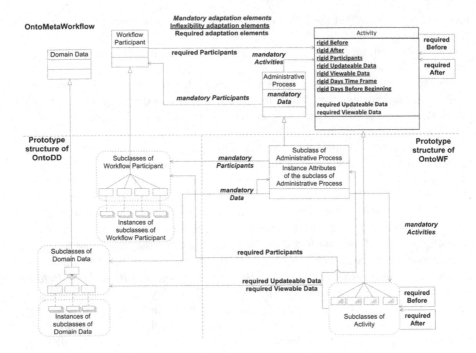

**Fig. 3** Adaptation elements of OntoMetaWorkflow

1. Identifying which activities should be mandatory in any possible hierarchical adaptation. All of them must be included in the *Mandatory Activities* relationship. The initial and the final activity, at least, must be mandatory.
2. Stablishing the degree of adaptability of the position of every activity inside the workflow by means of the attributes *Rigid After* and *Rigid Before*, and the relationships *Required After* and *Required Before*.
3. Specifying optional adaptation restrictions for every activity related to the involved participants (*Rigid Participants* attribute and *Required Participants* relationship), the required data (*Rigid Updateable Data* attribute, *Required Updateable Data* relationship, *Rigid Visible Data* attribute, *Required Visible Data* relationship) and the time constraints considered (*Rigid Days Time Frame* or *Rigid Days Before Beginning* attributes).

The result of applying this method must be a workflow correctly specified using *OntoMetaWorkflow* that is also an adaptable workflow.

Moreover, it should be pointed out that, although the adaptation elements are used only in the *OntoWF* ontology, also involve the *OntoDD* ontology. On the one hand, it is mandatory that the participants included in the *Mandatory Participants* relationship must be in the *OntoDD* ontology of the adapted workflow. On the other hand, it is also mandatory that the domain data included in the *Mandatory Data* relationship must be in the *OntoDD* ontology of the adapted workflow.

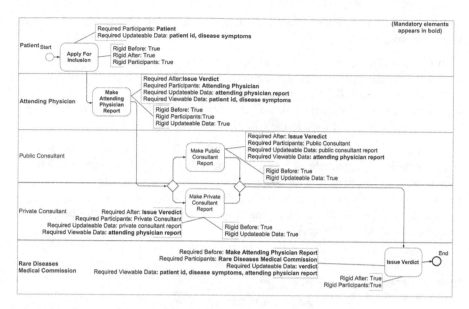

**Fig. 4** Specification of the adaptation restrictions in the inclusion process

Regarding our illustrative example, Fig. 4 shows the adaptation restrictions considered for that workflow. Due to the great number of restrictions, only the most illustrative ones are explained. Basically, the first activity, the second one and the last one are mandatory but it may be possible to remove the *Make Public Consultant Report* activity or the *Make Private Consultant Report* activity or even both. It is also worthy to note that the first activity and the last one allow adding new fields to fill in because they haven't set the *Rigid Updateable Data* attribute as true. However, the rest of the activities do not allow this choice in any possible adaptation. Finally, it is not possible to change the type of participants who can carry out every activity because all of them have set the *Rigid Participant* attribute as true.

## 2.3   Third Stage: Adaptation

For this stage, in first place the HAM establish the formal definition of an adapted workflow. So, an adapted workflow will be a workflow correctly specified using *OntoMetaWorkflow* that satisfy a set of implicit and explicit adaptation restrictions with respect to a given adaptable workflow.

On the one hand, the implicit restrictions do not depend on the adaptation elements. On the other hand, the explicit restrictions are related to the values set in the adaptation elements of the adaptable workflow.

In summary, a workflow will be a hierarchically adapted workflow from an adaptable workflow if:

- It is a workflow correctly specified using *OntoMetaWorkflow*.
- All the mandatory activities, participants, domain data and process properties of the adaptable workflow are in the adapted workflow.
- All the activities, mandatory or not, included in the adapted workflow, satisfy the restrictions established in their *Rigid* and *Required* attributes.

In order to specify correctly adapted workflows from an adaptable workflow, HAM provides 20 hierarchical adaptation operations, listed in Table 1. Those operations may be applied on an adaptable workflow to get the adapted workflow required. These operations use the basic modification operations of the first stage but adding a set of use restrictions that depend on the values of the adaptation elements of the adaptable workflow.

| **Table 1** Hierarchical adaptation operations | Operation |
| --- | --- |
| | Adaptation 1. Add New Activity |
| | Adaptation 2. Remove Activity |
| | Adaptation 3. Add New Workflow Participant |
| | Adaptation 4. Remove Workflow Participant |
| | Adaptation 5. Add New Domain Data |
| | Adaptation 6. Remove Domain Data |
| | Adaptation 7. Add New Process Property |
| | Adaptation 8. Remove Process Property |
| | Adaptation 9. Add Workflow Participant to Activity |
| | Adaptation 10. Remove Workflow Participant from Activity |
| | Adaptation 11. Add Domain Data to Select Class of Domain Data of Activity |
| | Adaptation 12. Remove Domain Data from Select Class of Domain Data of Activity |
| | Adaptation 13. Add Process Attribute to Fill In Instance Attributes of Process of Activity |
| | Adaptation 14. Remove Process Attribute from Fill In Instance Attributes of Process of Activity |
| | Adaptation 15. Add Domain Data to Show Class of Domain Data of Activity |
| | Adaptation 16. Remove Domain Data from Show Class of Domain Data of Activity |
| | Adaptation 17. Add Process Attribute to Show Instance Attributes of Process of Activity |
| | Adaptation 18. Remove Process Attribute from Show Instance Attributes of Process of Activity |
| | Adaptation 19. Reduce Days Time Frame of Activity |
| | Adaptation 20. Increase Days Before Beginning of Activity |

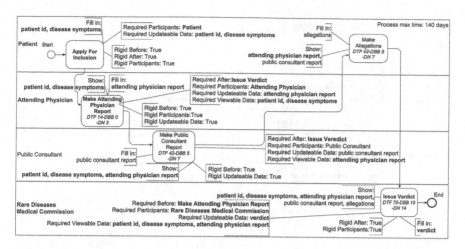

**Fig. 5** Adapted inclusion process

In the Rare Disease example, it may be possible for a Spanish region to apply the *Remove Activity* operation on the *Make Private Consultant Report* activity because the defined restrictions are satisfied. It may also be possible the incorporation of a new activity that allows patients to make new allegations on the diagnostic reports before the final verdict by using the *Add New Activity* operation. In Fig. 5 a process with these adaptations is shown.

## 2.4 Fourth Stage: Propagation

For this last stage, the HAM provides 60 hierarchical propagation operations that allow propagating the changes of an adaptable workflow to its adapted workflows. These operations are composed of two kinds of actions, firstly, the actions to change correctly the adaptable workflow and, secondly, the actions to propagate correctly the changes to the adapted workflows. These operations guarantee both the adaptable workflow and its adapted workflow will retain their status after applying them. These operations are not listed and nor explained in this work for the sake of brevity.

Regarding to the rare disease example, these operations may serve, firstly, to change the national adaptable workflow if the regulation that rules the process is changed and, secondly, to propagate those changes to the adapted workflows of the different regions (change synchronization). So, for example, if the national regulation changes the restrictions of the national process to state that *Issue Verdict* activity should always follow *Make Public Consultant Report* activity or *Make Private Consultant Report* activity, it would be necessary to apply the *Set Rigid After of Activity as True* operation on the two former activities. The application of

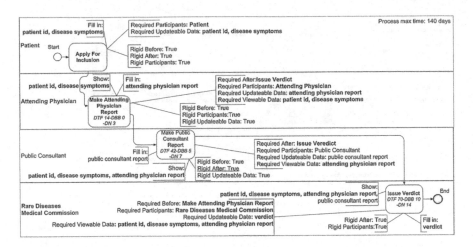

**Fig. 6** Adapted process after the propagation of the change

this operation would imply to remove the *Make Allegations* activity added in the stage three to the adapted workflow as can be seen in Fig. 6.

# 3   Related Works

The Hierarchical Adaptation Problem suggests the review of approaches dealing with workflow inheritance and specialization. A summary of the literature review performed is presented next.

One of the first approaches was named *Maximal Execution Set Semantics* [9–11]. Basically, it proposes to define a generic process as an abstract process containing all the different possible variations of a workflow. Then every workflow adaptation can be conceived as a specialization of such process. From a practical point of view, this approach cannot be applied to deal with the HAP, mainly because that implies to know every possible adaptation scenario beforehand.

One of the most well-known approaches is van der Aalst [12–14], named *Workflow Inheritance approach*. It is focused on the migration of running instances of a modified workflow. A workflow is considered a specialization if a new activity is added to the original workflow and its behavior remains unaltered when such activity is hidden or blocked. This approach is then focused in runtime, while the HAP should be resolved on definition time.

Wyner and Lee [15] proposed an interesting extension of the *Workflow Inheritance* approach best suited to deal with HAP. The authors introduced the concept of "frozen" elements that constrains the space of possible extensions of the original workflow. The HAP solution method (HAM) proposed herein extends that concept in the sense that different restriction levels can be established during original workflow design. The HAM provides the engineer with the necessary features (1) to set the required activities, data and participants in any possible adaptation of the original workflow; (2) to indicate the original workflow characteristics that should remain unaltered in any possible adaptation; and (3) to indicate the original workflow characteristics that should appear in any possible adaptation but open to modification. As Wyner and Lee [15] points out, the main issue to apply those ideas is the limited expressiveness of traditional workflow specification languages, as WF-net. That is the rationale behind the use of ontologies why the HAM, instead of common workflow languages, to represent administrative processes.

Schrefl and Stumptner [16], inspired by the concept of object life-cycle, define a specialization by means of the concepts of subnet, observation consistency and invocation consistency. The main objective of that approach is to keep the substitutability of the workflows, i.e. the original workflow may be seamlessly substituted by the adapted workflow and vice versa. That property, though interesting, is not always a main concern on the definition of administrative processes. Such kind of processes is often adapted to change the type of data required (or produced) or to change the type of their participants. And those adaptations may derive on not interchangeable workflows.

Other authors [17, 18] use the concept of non-monotonic inheritance as the base for their approach of process specialization. The concept of non-monotonic inheritance has also been considered in the HAM, although somewhat limited by the adaptation restrictions defined for every workflow.

Choppy et al. [19] define a process specialization according to its activities and the partial order they define to specify a concrete runtime path, called a process run. Their concept of partial order has also been introduced into the HAM. The generic workflow designer can indicate which activities should precede (or succeed) a concrete activity.

In conclusion, as far as we know, none of the reviewed approaches may be suitable to solve the Hierarchical Adaptation Problem. All of them are just focused on behavioral aspects and they are not concerned about data and participant adaptation issues. Most of them specified a set of predefined adaptation rules so the designer has not the possibility to define a customized specialization based on the concrete domain of the process. And, finally, none of them specify how to keep in sync the different adapted workflows with the original (generic) workflow when changes are introduced into the generic workflow.

## 4 Conclusions

The Hierarchical Adaptation Method has been presented in this paper to solve the Hierarchical Adaptation Problem. This problem arises in healthcare institutions whose processes are often defined by a higher-level entity (regional or national governments, the WHO...). It happens when it is necessary to adapt administrative workflows from the higher levels of the organizations to the particular conditions of the lower levels where they will be used, but satisfying the restrictions established in the higher levels.

As a result of the study of the literature, it can be argued that, as far as we know, this problem has been mainly addressed using the experience and intuition of the engineers responsible for solving them without the support of any formal systematic method. The Hierarchical Adaptation Method has been specifically proposed to cover that necessity.

This method takes advantage of the benefits of specifying workflows by means of ontologies using the *OntoMetaWorkflow* ontology. So, it proposes a formal way to specify the adaptation restrictions of the administrative workflows together with the operations needed to adapt them to the particular characteristics of every application case, complying with these adaptation restrictions. Furthermore, this method also provides the operations needed to propagate every possible change in the generic workflows to their adapted versions. It is important to note that, using this method, the restrictions that must meet a generic workflow and their adapted versions will be determined by the law or regulation that rules the process, and not by a previous rigid definition of adaptation that does not take into account the particular characteristics of every process. Thus, the Hierarchical Adaptation Method solves the Hierarchical Adaptation Problem providing a flexible adaptation method.

Two software tools[2] have been implemented in order to validate the approach in real scenarios; *WEAPON Designer*, which allows workflow designers to specify graphically an administrative workflow in *OntoDD* and *OntoWF* ontologies using *OntoMetaWorkflow*, and *WEAPON Manager*, a generic web application that manages the administrative workflows represented in the *OntoWF* and *OntoDD* ontologies by means of web forms. Until now, these tools have been applied on simulated scenarios of banking or healthing. The initial results have been successful. So, as main line of future work, its integration on real Bank or Health Information Systems is planned. Additionally, new software tools are currently under development to provide the engineer with a complete suite to assist with the application of the method.

# References

1. Feldman, M.S., Khademian, A.M.: Managing for inclusion: balancing control and participation. Int. Public Manag. J. **3**, 149–167 (2000)
2. Moore, J., Stader, J., Macintosh, A., Casson-du Mont, A., Chung, P.: Intelligent task management support for new product development in the chemical process industries. In: 6th International Product Development Management Conference (PDM 99), pp. 787–796, Cambridge, UK (1999)

---

[2]These software tools are available in http://uex.be/weapon.

3. Hollingsworth, D.: The Workflow Reference Model Document Number TC00-1003 Document Status—Issue 1.1., Winchester, UK (1995)
4. McReady, S.: There is more than one kind of Workflow Software (1992)
5. Georgakopoulos, D., Hornick, M., Sheth, A.: An overview of workflow management: from process modeling to workflow automation infrastructure. Distrib. Parallel Databases 3, 119–153 (1995)
6. Alonso, G., Agrawal, D., Abbadi, A.E., Mohan, C.: Functionality and limitations of current workflow management systems. IEEE Expert Intell. Syst. Appl. 12, 1–25 (1997)
7. Prieto, Á.E., Lozano-Tello, A.: Use of ontologies as representation support of workflows oriented to administrative management. J. Netw. Syst. Manag. 17, 309–325 (2009)
8. Prieto, A.E., Lozano-Tello, A.: Defining reusable administrative processes using a generic ontology. Int. J. Softw. Eng. Knowl. Eng. 22, 243–264 (2012)
9. Wyner, G.M., Lee, J.: Applying specialization to process models. In: Proceedings of the Conference on Computer Systems, pp. 290–301 (1995)
10. Malone, T.W., Crowston, K., Lee, J., Pentland, B., Dellarocas, C., Wyner, G.M., Quimby, J., Osborn, C.S., Bernstein, A., Herman, G., Klein, M., O'Donnell, E.: Tools for inventing organizations: Toward a handbook of organizational processes. Manage. Sci. 45, 425–443 (1999)
11. Lee, J., Wyner, G.M.: Defining specialization for dataflow diagrams. Inf. Syst. 28, 651–671 (2003)
12. Van Der Aalst, W.M.P., Basten, T.: Life-cycle inheritance: a Petri-Net-based approach. In: Proceedings of the 18th International Conference on Application and Theory of Petri Nets, pp. 62–81. Springer, London (1997)
13. Van Der Aalst, W.M.P., Basten, T.: Inheritance of workflows: an approach to tackling problems related to change. Theor. Comput. Sci. 270, 125–203 (2002)
14. Van Der Aalst, W.M.P.: Inheritance of business processes: a journey visiting four notorious problems. In: Ehrig, H., Reisig, W., Rozenberg, G., Weber, H. (eds.) Petri Net Technology for Communication-Based Systems. Lecture Notes in Computer Science, pp. 383–408. Springer, Berlin (2003)
15. Wyner, G.M., Lee, J.: Applying specialization to Petri Nets: implications for workflow design. In: Bussler, C.J., Haller, A. (eds.) Business Process Management Workshops. BPM 2005 International Workshops, BPI, BPD, ENEI, BPRM, WSCOBPM, BPS, Nancy, France, 5 Sept 2005. Revised Selected Papers, pp. 432–443. Springer, Berlin (2005)
16. Schrefl, M., Stumptner, M.: Behavior-consistent specialization of object life cycles. ACM Trans. Softw. Eng. Methodol. 11, 92–148 (2002)
17. Bernstein, A., Grosof, B.N.: Beyond Monotonic Inheritance: Towards Semantic Web Process Ontologies (2003)
18. Ferndriger, S., Bernstein, A., Dong, J.S., Feng, Y., Li, Y.-F., Hunter, J.: Enhancing semantic web services with inheritance. In: Proceedings of the 7th International Conference on the Semantic Web, pp. 162–177. Springer, Berlin (2008)
19. Choppy, C., Desel, J., Petrucci, L.: Specialisation and generalisation of processes. In: Proceedings of the Workshop on Petri Nets and Software Engineering (PNSE'11), Newcastle, UK, pp. 109–123. CEUR-WS (2011)

# A Monitoring Infrastructure for the Quality Assessment of Cloud Services

Priscila Cedillo, Javier Gonzalez-Huerta, Silvia Abrahao
and Emilio Insfran

**Abstract** Service Level Agreements (SLAs) specify the strict terms under which cloud services must be provided. The assessment of the quality of services being provided is critical for both clients and service providers. In this context, stakeholders must be capable of monitoring services delivered as Software as a Service (SaaS) at runtime and of reporting any eventual non-compliance with SLAs in a comprehensive and flexible manner. In this paper, we present the definition of an SLA compliance monitoring infrastructure, which is based on the use of models@run.time, its main components and artifacts, and the interactions among them. We place emphasis on the configuration of the artifacts that will enable the monitoring, and we present a prototype that can be used to perform this monitoring. The feasibility of our proposal is illustrated by means of a case study, which shows the use of the components and artifacts in the infrastructure and the configuration of a specific plan with which to monitor the services deployed on the Microsoft Azure© platform.

A prior version of this paper has been published in the ISD2015 Proceedings (http://aisel.aisnet.org/isd2014/proceedings2015/).

P. Cedillo · S. Abrahao · E. Insfran
Department of Computer Systems and Computation,
Universitat Politècnica de València, Valencia, Spain
e-mail: sabrahao@dsic.upv.es

E. Insfran
e-mail: einsfran@dsic.upv.es

P. Cedillo (✉)
Department of Computer Science, Faculty of Engineering,
University of Cuenca, Cuenca, Ecuador
e-mail: priscila.cedillo@ucuenca.edu.ec; icedillo@dsic.upv.es

J. Gonzalez-Huerta
Département d'Informatique, Université du Québec à Montréal,
Montreal, Canada
e-mail: gonzalez_huerta.javier@uqam.ca

© Springer International Publishing Switzerland 2016
D. Vogel et al. (eds.), *Transforming Healthcare Through Information Systems*,
Lecture Notes in Information Systems and Organisation 17,
DOI 10.1007/978-3-319-30133-4_2

17

**Keywords** Model driven engineering · Models@run.time · Quality assessment · Cloud services · Service level agreements · Software as a service

# 1 Introduction

Software as a Service (SaaS) has emerged as a software deployment model in recent years that makes software available entirely through the use of a web browser, while hiding the details regarding where the software is hosted or its underlying architecture [1]. SaaS is increasingly being used by web-based applications owing the benefits it provides for both users and service providers [2]. The terms under which a SaaS application is provided must be expressed by using Service Level Agreements (SLAs). Each service is typically accompanied by an SLA that defines the minimal guarantees that the cloud provider offers to its customers [3] (e.g. ensuring the availability of a service at least 99.5 % of the time). Service providers are becoming interested in monitoring cloud services in order to assess compliance with the SLA, thus avoiding possible penalizations and improving service quality [4]. On the customer side, service monitoring provides information and Key Performance Indicators (KPIs) that are useful in the decision-making process [5].

Traditional monitoring technologies are restricted to static and homogeneous environments, and cannot therefore be appropriately applied to cloud environments [6]. Cloud computing has led to the emergence of new issues, challenges, and needs as regards measuring quality (e.g. elasticity, scalability, adaptability, timeliness) [5]. Moreover, when compared with other distributed systems such as Grid Computing, the monitoring of a cloud is more complex because of the differences in both the trust model and the view of resources/services presented to the user [7], in addition to the presence of multiple layers and service paradigms [5]. Unfortunately, existing cloud and general purpose monitoring solutions have several limitations, as reported by Muller et al. [8]: the SLAs they support are not sufficiently expressive to model real-world scenarios. They couple the monitoring configuration with a given SLA specification, the explanations of the violations are difficult to understand and even potentially inaccurate, and some proposals either do not provide an architecture or the cohesion of their elements is low. Furthermore, it is important to have flexible quality monitoring infrastructures that will allow service providers to modify the non-functional requirements (NFRs) to be monitored, based on SLAs variations.

We believe that Model Driven Engineering (MDE) may be a solution as regards providing the flexibility required to monitor infrastructures. However, establishing all the NFRs to be monitored when designing the monitoring infrastructure is not always possible (e.g., owing to SLA renegotiations, the addition of new NFRs to be monitored, changes in the cloud platform). In this context, Baresi and Ghezzi [9] advocate that future software engineering research should be focused on providing software with intelligent support at runtime, thus breaking across the current rigid boundary between development-time and runtime. It is therefore necessary to define approaches that will allow cloud services to be monitored and will also permit the addition of new requirements or the modification of existing ones at runtime without interrupting the service execution. This challenge can be confronted by using models@run.time [9]. A model@run.time is employed at runtime in a system and its encoding enables its processing at runtime [10]. Besides, a model@run.time is causally-connected to the running system, meaning that a change in this model triggers a corresponding change in the running system and/or vice versa [10].

In a previous paper, we presented the definition of a monitoring process for cloud services by using models@run.time [11], in which we established the tasks involved in the monitoring process. In this paper, we extend that work by presenting the monitoring infrastructure that using models@run.time is able to: (i) retrieve data from the cloud services during their execution; (ii) calculate derived metrics based on these data; and (iii) report any eventual SLA violations. The contribution of this paper is therefore the definition of a monitoring infrastructure, its main components and the artifacts used by the Monitoring Configurator (i.e., quality meta-models with which to generate the Requirements Quality Model, the SaaS Quality Model and the Runtime Quality Model), along with the interactions among them. The feasibility of our proposal is illustrated through a case study, which shows the use of the components and artifacts involved in the infrastructure and the configuration of a specific monitoring plan for the Microsoft Azure© platform.

The paper is structured as follows: Sect. 2 discusses the existing solutions. Section 3 presents the monitoring infrastructure, its components and artifacts. Section 4 presents a case study. Finally, Sect. 5 presents the conclusions and future work.

## 2  Related Work

Several studies whose aim has been to analyze the monitoring tools and approaches that are available (e.g., [5, 12]) and their weaknesses and needs have appeared over the last few years. Fatema et al. [12] report the results of a survey in which they analyze cloud and general purpose monitoring tools. They identify practical capabilities that an ideal monitoring tool should possess in order to fulfill the objectives of both cloud providers and customers in different cloud operational areas. They conclude that most general purpose monitoring tools were not designed with the cloud in mind, signifying that most monitoring capabilities (e.g. multi-tenancy, scalability, non-intrusiveness) are improved using cloud based monitoring tools. However, one of the drawbacks of cloud monitoring tools is their portability. This reinforces the fact that many cloud specific monitoring tools are commercial and vendor dependent, which makes the tools less flexible and portable and means that their results are neither extensible nor comparable to other platforms. Aceto et al. [5] analyze and discuss the properties of a monitoring system for the cloud. They conclude that cloud monitoring tools should have quality characteristics (e.g., scalability, elasticity, adaptability) that will enable them to tackle the challenges that cloud monitoring implies. However, they also conclude that current solutions still require considerable effort if desirable characteristics are to be attained.

Many cloud providers offer their customers the ability to monitor cloud services using monitoring tools available for CPU, storage and network [13]. These tools are closely integrated with their own cloud solutions. They are only concerned with monitoring quality attributes for the hardware resources (CPU, storage, and network) and lack the ability to monitor application-specific QoS parameters and SLA requirements (i.e., latency, performance). In addition, the majority of commercial tools (e.g., CloudWatch, LogicMonitor) are not sufficiently flexible to allow service providers to extend the QoS parameters provided to monitor the fulfillment of SLAs.

Various approaches have also been proposed in academic environments. For instance, Emeakaroha et al. [14] propose an application monitoring architecture named Cloud Application SLA violation Detection architecture (CASViD). This architecture monitors and detects SLA violations on the application layer, and includes tools for resource allocation, scheduling, and deployment. Although their approach provides a good solution, it does not have a flexible means to change the NFRs and metrics to be monitored at runtime. Katsaros et al. [15] present a monitoring system that facilitates on-the-fly self-configuration in terms of both the monitoring time and the monitoring parameters. They propose the use of scripts to collect data; however, they do not specify how NFRs are matched with raw data gathered from scripts and how they interact with cloud services. Müller et al. [8] designed and implemented SALMonADA, a service-based system with which to monitor and analyze SLAs in order to provide an explanation of violations. They describe SLAs using a Monitoring Management Document (MMD) to be consumed by the monitoring infrastructure; however, the platform does not support those users who wish to choose alternative means to measure quality requirements. Smit et al. [16] present and implement an architecture using stream processing to provide service monitoring. They emphasize that their infrastructure is intended be used to monitor hybrid clouds and two tiered cloud architectures working on streaming data. The possibility of gathering information therefore depends on the information that can be provided by other solutions. Montes et al. [17] propose a cloud monitoring taxonomy, which is used as the basis to define a layered cloud monitoring architecture. They implement GMonE, a general-purpose cloud monitoring tool, which is claimed to cover all aspects of cloud monitoring by specifically addressing the needs of modern cloud infrastructures. Similarly, Povedano-Molina et al. [18] propose DARGOS, a distributed architecture for resource management and monitoring in clouds, which ensures an accurate measurement of physical and virtual resources in the cloud in an attempt to keep overheads down. However, the latter two approaches confront the provision of only physical and virtual resources and do not emphasize the specific quality aspects of SaaS. In summary, to the best of our knowledge commercial tools are mostly tightly coupled with certain cloud platforms, support the monitoring of specific NFRs, and have pre-established low-level metrics; they are therefore not sufficiently versatile to support the modification of NFRs or the customization of their operationalizations[1] at runtime. There are other proposals that

---

[1]Operationalizing a measure consists of establishing a mapping between its generic description and the concepts represented in the software artifacts to be measured [30].

allow the verification of SLA compliance, but they are not enough flexible to support different operationalizations according to the specific cloud platform involved.

## 3 Monitoring Infrastructure

In this section, we present the *Monitoring Infrastructure* that has been designed to support the monitoring process defined in Cedillo et al. [11] (see Fig. 1). This infrastructure allows: (i) the specification and configuration of NFRs to be monitored; (ii) an interaction with cloud services to assess their quality at runtime; (iii) and the generation of reports containing any eventual SLA violations. In order to achieve these goals and provide the required degree of flexibility when defining NFR metrics, in addition to supporting different means to gather information from cloud services, we have defined a set of components and artifacts that conform to the monitoring infrastructure by using models@run.time. The solution is oriented to be applied in any platform, a detailed instantiation of the middleware to a defined platform is presented in Cedillo et al. [19].

The Monitoring Infrastructure has two main components: the *Monitoring Configurator* and the *Monitoring and Analysis Middleware*. The Monitoring Configurator uses the *Monitoring Requirements Model* and the *SaaS Quality Model* to configure the monitoring of services and obtain the *Runtime Quality Model*. The *Monitoring and Analysis Middleware* uses this Runtime Quality Model and relies on two engines: the *Measurements Engine,* which permits cloud service monitoring through the use of the raw service quality data gathered from cloud services and takes the measurements, and the *Analysis Engine,* which compares the expected values with the monitored values and can generate the SLA violations report. The details of each process and artifact are detailed in the following subsections.

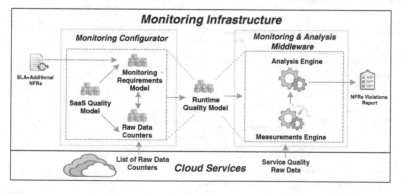

**Fig. 1** Monitoring infrastructure

## 3.1   Monitoring Configurator

The Monitoring Configurator is a component of the Monitoring Infrastructure (see Fig. 1) and has a front-end which is used by stakeholders to configure the monitoring directives. It allows the high level NFRs to be monitored that are included in the Monitoring Requirements Model and the raw service quality data retrieved from cloud services to be matched. This matching is supported by the SaaS Quality Model, which acts as a guide that allows the selection of appropriate operationalizations for metrics. When the matching is done by stakeholders, the Runtime Quality Model is generated and can be consumed by the Monitoring and Analysis Middleware. A detailed description of the artifacts involved in the Monitoring Configurator and the interactions among them is shown below.

**Monitoring Requirements Model** This model specifies the NFRs to be monitored comprehensible way for the Monitoring Infrastructure, compliant with the WSLA Language Specification [20] to represent NFRs in a standardized manner. Moreover, in our solution, the model is extended to support additional NFRs that are not part of SLAs but which may be of interest to stakeholders. Figure 2 shows the monitoring requirements meta-model, which incorporates all the SLA sections. The SLA specifies the parties, divided into signatory parties and supporting parties. On the one hand, signatory parties, namely service provider and service customer, are assumed to "sign" the SLA, while on the other, supporting parties are sponsored by signatory parties to provide service measurements and audits. The meta-model includes the SLAParameter meta-class, which represents the NFRs to be monitored and the Metrics used to perform measurements. A Service Object is the abstraction of a service, whose quality characteristics and attributes are relevant as regards defining the SLA's terms. Characteristics and attributes are specified as

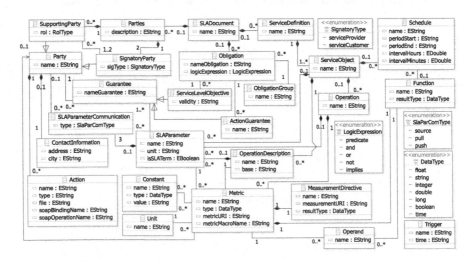

**Fig. 2**  Monitoring requirements meta-model

SLAParameters. Each SLAParameter can be measured by using metrics. The SLAParameter meta-class has an attribute named isSLATerm, which differentiates an SLA term from an NFR that is not included in the SLA. The Obligation meta-class contains two types of obligations: (i) a Service Level Objective, which is a guarantee of a particular state of SLA parameters in a given time period. (e.g. the average response time must be 5 ms) and (ii) The Action Guarantee, which specifies the provider's commitment to doing something in a specific situation [21] (e.g. if a violation of a guarantee occurs, a notification is sent specifying a penalty). The values used as thresholds are obtained from the Action Guarantee meta-class (e.g. the response time must be <0.7 unless the transaction rate is >1000). In this meta-model, a metric can be measured by using the formula agreed by the parties. A more detailed specification of the WSLA used to define the meta-classes, with examples, can be found in Ludwig et al. [20].

**SaaS Quality Model** This model is aligned with the ISO/IEC 25010 standard (SQuaRE) [21]. Figure 3 shows the meta-model supporting the SaaS Quality Model. This model allows the definition of the whole set of Characteristics, Sub-characteristics, Attributes, their Impact (i.e., the relationships among attributes), and Metrics that specify how NFRs should be measured to assess the quality of cloud services. Each metric can be operationalized in different ways. A metric Operationalization can be considered at different Cloud Levels (i.e., SaaS, PaaS, IaaS). This is useful owing to the fact that there are a number of quality requirements (e.g., scalability, elasticity, security) that need to be monitored for different levels of service provision [5]. Moreover, it is important to specify the stakeholder that will use the monitoring information; for example, for a service provider, it may be interesting to know the average number of users requesting a service at a particular time. The purpose of having perspectives associated with each operationalization is to express whether a given operationalization is stakeholder-specific. This information is useful during the processes of comparing, improving measurements, or choosing different formulas with which to measure each NFR. The DirectMetricOperationalization meta-class represents a measure of an attribute that does not depend upon any other measure, whereas the

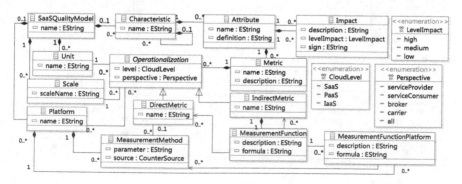

**Fig. 3** SaaS quality meta-model

IndirectMetricOperationalization meta-class represents measures that are derived from other DirectMetricOperationalizations or IndirectMetricOperationalizations. The Platform and MeasurementMethod meta-classes have been added to the SaaS Quality Model to maintain a list of raw platform dependent data counters to facilitate the retrieval of information from a specific platform. Finally, the meta-model includes particularities of each operationalization, such as the Unit meta-class, which expresses the magnitude related to a particular quantity. The Scale meta-class represents a set of values with continuous or discrete properties used to map the operationalization.

**Runtime Quality Model** This is a model@run.time, which specifies the monitoring requirements, metrics, operationalizations, and configurations that will be used during the monitoring. Lehmann et al. [22] argue that meta-models at runtime must provide modeling constructs that will enable the definition of: (a) A prescriptive part of the model, specifying what the system should be like; (b) A descriptive part of the model specifying what the system is like; (c) Valid model modifications of the descriptive parts, executable at runtime; (d) Valid model modifications of the prescriptive parts, executable at runtime; (e) Causal connection, which is in the form of an information flow between the model and the entity being monitored. Figure 4 shows the Runtime Quality Meta-model, which is an extension of the SaaS Quality Model. It has many of the meta-classes included in the SaaS Quality Model described previously, plus meta-classes that represent the prescriptive part, the descriptive part, and the characteristics of the cloud platform that allow the causal connection.

The CloudService meta-class also describes the service to be monitored. The prescriptive part of the model thus includes the *Threshold*, which is obtained from the obligations part of the SLA, or an AdditionalNFR threshold set by the

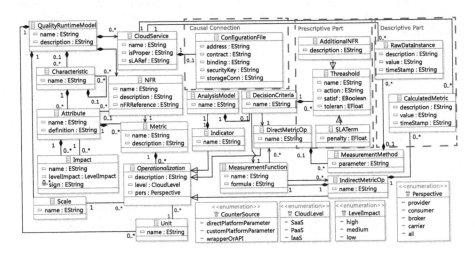

**Fig. 4** Runtime quality meta-model

stakeholder. The descriptive part of the model is formed of the RawDataInstance meta-class, which contains the values captured directly from the cloud, and the CalculatedMetric meta-class, which contains the measurement results of the calculated metrics. The ConfigurationFile meta-class contains specific information for each platform that allows an interaction to take place between the monitoring infrastructure and the cloud service. It can therefore be considered as the class that is used to attain the causal connection between the monitoring infrastructure and services when a change needs to be reflected. Finally, the Indicator meta-class represents a measure that is derived from the other measures using an Analysis Model as a measurement approach [23]. In conclusion, the Runtime Quality Model allows our proposal to obtain the desirable characteristics related to flexibility and maintainability, since changes in the Runtime Quality Model can be easily reflected in the monitoring infrastructure.

**Interaction Among Models** Figure 5 shows the interactions among the models. The first interaction (1) occurs between the SaaS Quality Model and the Monitoring Requirements Model. Stakeholders can use the SaaS Quality Model, which contains a standardized classification of characteristics, sub-characteristics, metrics, and attributes, as support in order to define the Monitoring Requirements Model. The second interaction (2) then occurs between the Monitoring Requirements Model and the Runtime Quality Model. Here, the stakeholder uses the Monitoring Configurator Interface to capture the NFRs and metrics included in the Monitoring Requirements Model to define the Runtime Quality Model. Finally, the third interaction (3) occurs between the Runtime Quality Model and the SaaS Quality Model. This interaction allows the means used to gather information from cloud services to be specified. In this scenario, the SaaS Quality Model is useful as regards matching the high level attributes contained in the Monitoring Requirements Model with raw service quality data. Here, the SaaS Quality Model

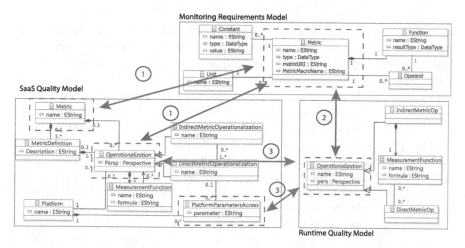

**Fig. 5** Interaction among models

enables a choice to be made from among many equivalent operationalizations with different measurement methods, thus providing our approach with flexibility.

## 3.2   Monitoring and Analysis Middleware

The Monitoring and Analysis Middleware consists of the Measurements Engine, which uses the Runtime Quality Model obtained as result of the configuration as input, and this applies metrics with which to measure the quality of services. There is also the Analysis Engine, which permits the analysis of quality and reports SLA violations. A description of the Monitoring Middleware components has been addressed in Cedillo et al. [19].

# 4   Case Study

An exploratory case study was performed following the guidelines presented in Runeson et al. [24] in order to analyze the feasibility of the configuration task. The stages of the case study are: design, preparation, collection of data, and analysis of data, each of which is explained below. In this case study, we have used a metric to illustrate the configuration task. In Cedillo et al. [19], it can be found other examples to have a better idea about the configuration and application of other NFRs to this solution.

## 4.1   Design of the Case Study

The case study was designed by considering the five components proposed in Runeson et al. [24]: purpose of the study, underlying conceptual framework, research questions to be addressed, sampling strategy, and methods employed.

The purpose of this case study is to analyze the feasibility of configuring the monitoring of services by means of the Monitoring Configurator, and to use these configurations to generate the Runtime Quality Model. The Monitoring and Analysis Middleware will take this model as input to monitor the cloud services. The conceptual framework that links the phenomena to be studied is based on the Monitoring Process [11] and an infrastructure that supports this process (i.e., components, artifacts). The research questions to be addressed are: (a) is the strategy of configuring and matching the NFRs with quality raw data retrieved from cloud services to obtain the desired monitoring information useable and effective?; (b) what are the limitations of the monitoring configurator?

Here, the sampling strategy is based on monitoring configuration tests carried out by a subject who is an IT professional with programming skills and who has been working as a Cloud Provider Service Specialist for two years. In accordance with Lethbridge et al. [25], we have applied the second degree of data collection techniques, in which the researcher directly collects raw data without interacting with the subject during the data collection.

In order to collect the monitoring information, we developed a prototype of the Monitoring and Analysis Middleware that allows the collection of raw data through the use of the Runtime Quality Model generated in the configuration task. The monitoring configuration was carried out as follows: the subject used the Monitoring Requirements Model to match NFRs with quality parameters and instructions that gather data from a service running in the cloud. The technique used to obtain feedback regarding the feasibility of the monitoring configuration performed was an analysis of the monitoring results obtained using a prototype of the Monitoring Engine to obtain the data needed to prove whether the values gathered were those expected by the subject.

## 4.2 Preparation of the Case Study

The context of this case study, was a test scenario in which the subject carried out the monitoring configuration. The SaaS Quality Model was used to support the matching between the NFRs to be monitored and the platform information. Once this information had been matched, it was possible to generate the Runtime Quality Model, which was then used by the Monitoring and Analysis Middleware to gather, measure and analyze quality data obtained from cloud services. The services used in this case study were implemented in compliance with an Open Reference Case (ORC) proposed in Ludwig et al. [20], which was used as an open source demonstrator to highlight the achievements of the European research project SLA@SOI. The ORC is an extension of the CoCoMe implementation [26], which provides a service oriented retail solution that can be used in a supermarket trading system to handle the sales and stocking process [27]. The set of services defined by ORC was deployed as a SaaS on the Microsoft Azure© platform. We considered the actions (i.e., create, read, update, and delete operations) related to the inventory service and the sales service. The objective was to configure the monitoring infrastructure in order to perform quality evaluations of cloud services. The NFRs to be monitored were reliability and latency.

Figure 6 presents an excerpt of an instance of the Monitoring Requirements. It shows the service, its operations (e.g. NewItemInventory) and the NFRs (SLAParameters). The NFRs to be monitored are the *reliability* and *latency* of the inventory and sales cloud services. *Reliability* is defined as "*the ability of an item to perform a required function under stated conditions for a stated time period*" [28]. Customers and suppliers often measure service reliability as Defective operations Per Million attempts (DPM) [29]. In this case study, the SLA term included the following clause: "the service could have a maximum of ten defective operations per million" (i.e., "99.999 % service reliability"). *Service latency* was, meanwhile,

**Fig. 6** Monitoring
requirements model instance
excerpt

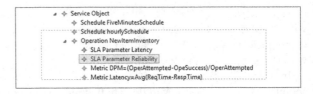

defined as "*the time that has elapsed between a request and the corresponding response*" [29], and thus "the maximum service latency is 130 ms". The *Monitoring Requirements Model* includes the DPM metric which measures reliability. It was then necessary to select the DPM equivalent operationalization, which allows the measurement of the reliability NFR in cloud services deployed on the Microsoft Azure © platform. Our SaaS Quality Model contains three equivalent metric operationalizations (i.e. DPM1, DPM2, and DPM3). The subject select one of them depending on the Monitoring Requirements Model and the Raw Service Quality Data to be retrieved.

The operationalizations included in our SaaS Quality Model to calculate DPM are:

$$DPM\ 1 = \frac{OperationsAttempted - Operations\ Successful}{Operations\ Attempted} \times 10^6 \qquad (1)$$

$$DPM\ 2 = \frac{Operations\ Failed}{Operations\ Attempted} \times 10^6 \qquad (2)$$

$$DPM\ 2 = \frac{Operations\ Failed}{OperationsSuccessful + OperationsFailed} \times 10^6 \qquad (3)$$

The subject can select an equivalent operationalization by considering the advantages and disadvantages of the selection (e.g. overheads). Once the Runtime Quality Model has been generated, the Monitoring and Analysis Middleware can collect information, measure data, and report SLA violations. Here, data is captured by using the Azure Diagnostics Service. However, this could change depending on the facilities of each cloud platform. Here, the subject can use one of the three equations (1)–(3) to match that selection with Diagnostics counters. Finally, the matched formula was used for the Monitoring and Analysis Middleware using Diagnostics counters.

## 4.3   Collection of Data

The data was collected in two stages: (1) when the subject carried out the configurations depending on the NFRs and matched these NFRs with raw platform-specific data counters to generate the Runtime Quality Model using the

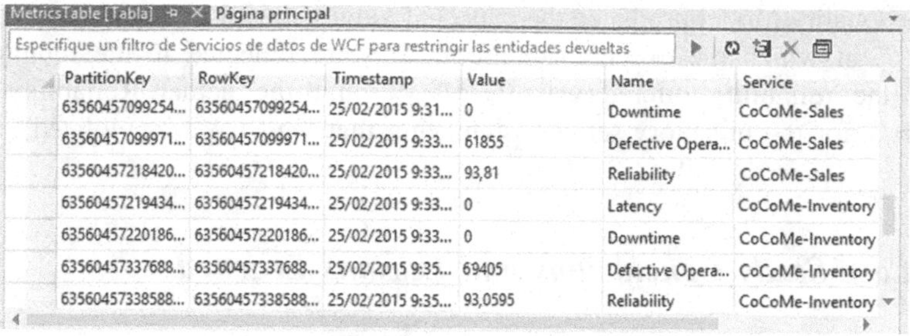

| MetricsTable [Tabla] | | Página principal | | | | |

| | Especifique un filtro de Servicios de datos de WCF para restringir las entidades devueltas | | | | | |
|---|---|---|---|---|---|---|
| PartitionKey | RowKey | Timestamp | Value | | Name | Service |
| 63560457099254... | 63560457099254... | 25/02/2015 9:31... | 0 | | Downtime | CoCoMe-Sales |
| 63560457099971... | 63560457099971... | 25/02/2015 9:33... | 61855 | | Defective Opera... | CoCoMe-Sales |
| 63560457218420... | 63560457218420... | 25/02/2015 9:33... | 93,81 | | Reliability | CoCoMe-Sales |
| 63560457219434... | 63560457219434... | 25/02/2015 9:33... | 0 | | Latency | CoCoMe-Inventory |
| 63560457220186... | 63560457220186... | 25/02/2015 9:33... | 0 | | Downtime | CoCoMe-Inventory |
| 63560457337688... | 63560457337688... | 25/02/2015 9:35... | 69405 | | Defective Opera... | CoCoMe-Inventory |
| 63560457338588... | 63560457338588... | 25/02/2015 9:35... | 93,0595 | | Reliability | CoCoMe-Inventory |

**Fig. 7** Metrics calculated by using the monitoring infrastructure

SaaS Quality Model; (2) when the monitoring engine gathered and measured information provided by cloud services based on the Runtime Quality Model. A prototype of the Monitoring and Analysis Middleware was implemented as a Microsoft Azure cloud service, which stores the results in a data base. Figure 7 shows the results with the calculated metrics.

## 4.4 Analysis of Data

The monitoring configuration was analyzed so as to address our research questions. The subject used the Monitoring Requirements Model, which contained the NFRs to be monitored, and their metrics and thresholds. The subject then matched the metrics with the appropriate operationalizations specific to the platform. In order to illustrate the process used to monitor the reliability, the other NFRs were monitored following analogous steps. The reliability threshold was 99.999 %, and we the considered operationalization (1) which was set up by matching formula (4) with the Azure Counters:

- RequestsTotal=@"\ASP.NET Applications(_Total_)\Requests Total"
- OperationsSuccessful=@"\ASP.NET Applications(_Total_)\Requests Succeeded"

$$DPM = \frac{RequestsTotal - RequestsSucceded}{RequestsTotal} \tag{4}$$

The Runtime Quality Model should include Formula (4). When checking whether the monitoring infrastructure would be able to monitor the behavior of the cloud services by using the runtime quality model, we intentionally introduced exceptions into the ORC services' source code to generate reliability and latency problems.

It was necessary to determine whether the configuration gathers the expected information from the cloud services by using the Runtime Quality Model and to find possible limitations or inaccurate results. Here, we have concluded that the

Runtime Quality Model produced the expected values shown in the table presented in Fig. 7, in which the exceptions introduced were reflected in the monitoring results (the reliability offered was 99.999 % and the actual Reliability was 93.0595 % for the inventory service, signifying that the SLA was violated).

## 4.5   Case Study Conclusions and Lessons Learned

With regard to the first research question stated for this case study, we provide support to help the configuration of NFRs to be monitored using our approach and that the configuration was effective as regards monitoring Azure cloud services. Moreover, the suitability of this approach is shown by the fact that it is feasible to use the Monitoring Configurator to match the NFRs included in the Monitoring Requirements Model with the raw service quality data gathered from the cloud service and provide the expected information. With regard to the second research question, the Monitoring Infrastructure is able to detect SLA violations from a wide range of NFRs. However, it is important to take into account that not all the NFRs can be monitored owing to the restriction of the infrastructure that provides the raw service quality data from the services. One solution to this issue would be to use wrappers for services in order to capture the information required in a customized manner, which constitutes one of the next steps in our research.

As lessons learned this case study has allowed us to observe the potentialities and limitations of our proposal. The monitoring configurator allows a wide variety of operationalizations and platform counters to be matched. However, it depends on the facilities used to provide raw service quality data. During the execution of the case study, several aspects related to how the configuration can be facilitated have been discovered. For example, the SaaS Quality Model provides a simple means to choose the operationalizations and it is possible to add operationalizations to the SaaS Quality Model, which represents a knowledge base that saves efforts and minimizes possible mistakes when the configuring task is being carried out.

## 5   Conclusions and Future Work

In this paper, we have presented a monitoring infrastructure for cloud services, which allows data to be retrieved from cloud services in order to calculate monitoring metrics and eventually report non-compliance with the SLA. The monitoring infrastructure uses the Runtime Quality Model, which is generated by using two additional models: the Monitoring Requirements Model and the SaaS Quality Model. The feasibility of the approach has been illustrated by means of a case study which shows the monitoring of services deployed on the Azure platform.

The use of models@run.time provides flexibility and eases maintainability when the SLA and additional NFRs to be monitored change. Moreover, the facility of changing the model and not the monitoring infrastructure makes it easier to operate and understand when they are not familiar with the middleware implementation.

As future work, we plan to deliver our Monitoring and Analysis Middleware in other platforms (e.g. Amazon AWS, Google) to be able to monitor and analyze services deployed in these platforms. We also plan to carry out a systematic review of the quality characteristics, sub-characteristics, attributes, and metrics of cloud services. The findings will be included in the SaaS Quality Model in order to study the monitoring mechanisms provided by other commonly used cloud platforms such as Google App Engine or Amazon AWS. Moreover, we plan to study generic means to encapsulate the raw data collected from the cloud services in order to obtain common interfaces for many platforms (e.g., APIs, proxies, plugins). Finally, we plan to improve the efficiency of the proposal by taking in account issues such as overheads, security, etc. and to empirically validate the approach using controlled experiments.

**Acknowledgments** This research has been supported by the Value@Cloud project (TIN2013-46300-R), Scholarship Program Senescyt-Ecuador, NSERC (Natural Sciences and Engineering Research Council of Canada) and Microsoft Azure for Research Award Program.

# References

1. Sriram, I., Khajeh-Hosseini, A.: Research agenda in cloud technologies. In: 1st ACM Symposium on Cloud Computing, SOCC, pp. 1–11 (2010)
2. Song, J., Han, F., Yan, Z., Liu, G., Zhu, Z.: A SaaSify tool for converting traditional web-based apps to SaaS application. In: 4th International Conference on Cloud Computing, CLOUD, pp. 396–403 (2011)
3. Baset, S.A.: Cloud SLAs: present and future. ACM SIGOPS Oper. Syst. **46**, 57–66 (2012)
4. Hassan, M., Song, B., Huh, E.-N.: A market-oriented dynamic collaborative cloud services platform. Ann. Telecommun. **65**, 669–688 (2010)
5. Aceto, G., Botta, A., de Donato, W., Pescapè, A.: Cloud monitoring: a survey. Comput. Netw. **57**, 2093–2115 (2013)
6. Shao, J., Wei, H., Wang, Q., Mei, H.: A runtime model based monitoring approach for cloud. In: International Conference on Cloud Computing (CLOUD), pp. 313–320 (2010)
7. Foster, I., Zhao, Y., Raicu, I., Lu, S.: Cloud computing and grid computing 360-degree compared. In: Grid Computing Environments Workshop (GCE 08), pp. 1–10 (2008)
8. Muller, C., Oriol, M., Franch, X., Marco, J., Resinas, M., Ruiz-Cortes, A., Rodriguez, M.: Comprehensive explanation of SLA violations at runtime. IEEE Trans. Serv. Comput. **7**, 168–183 (2014)
9. Baresi, L., Ghezzi, C.: The disappearing boundary between development-time and run-time. In: Workshop on the Future of Software Engineering Research FSE/SDP, pp. 17–22. ACM, USA (2010)
10. Giese, H., Bencomo, N., Pasquale, L., Ramirez, A., Inverardi, P., Wätzoldt, S., Clarke, S.: Living with Uncertainty in the Age of Runtime Models. http://dx.doi.org/10.1007/978-3-319-08915-7_3
11. Cedillo, P., Gonzalez-Huerta, J., Insfrán, E., Abrahao, S.: Towards monitoring cloud services using Models@run.time. In: Workshop on Models@run.time, MODELS, pp. 31–40, Spain (2014)

12. Fatema, K., Emeakaroha, V.C., Healy, P.D., Morrison, J.P., Lynn, T.: A survey of cloud monitoring tools: taxonomy, capabilities and objectives (2014)
13. Alhamazani, K., Ranjan, R., Mitra, K., Rabhi, F., Jayaraman, P.P., Khan, S.U., Guabtni, A., Bhatnagar, V.: An overview of the commercial cloud monitoring tools: research dimensions, design issues, and state-of-the-art. Computing, pp. 1–21 (2014)
14. Emeakaroha, V.C., Ferreto, T.C., Netto, M.A.S., Brandic, I., De Rose, C.A.F.: CASViD: application level monitoring for SLA violation detection in clouds. In: Computer Software and Applications Conference (COMPSAC), pp. 499–508 (2012)
15. Katsaros, G., Kousiouris, G., Gogouvitis, S.V., Kyriazis, D., Menychtas, A., Varvarigou, T.: A self-adaptive hierarchical monitoring mechanism for Clouds. J. Syst. Softw. **85**, 1029–1041 (2012)
16. Smit, M., Simmons, B., Litoiu, M.: Distributed, application-level monitoring for heterogeneous clouds using stream processing. Future Gener. Comput. Syst. **29**, 2103–2114 (2013)
17. Montes, J., Sánchez, A., Memishi, B., Pérez, M.S., Antoniu, G.: GMonE: a complete approach to cloud monitoring. Future Gener. Comput. Syst. **29**, 2026–2040 (2013)
18. Povedano-Molina, J., Lopez-Vega, J.M., Lopez-Soler, J.M., Corradi, A., Foschini, L.: DARGOS: a highly adaptable and scalable monitoring architecture for multi-tenant Clouds. Future Gener. Comput. Syst. **29**, 2041–2056 (2013)
19. Cedillo, P., Jimenez-Gomez, J., Abrahao, S., Insfran, E.: Towards a monitoring middleware for Cloud services. In: International Conference on Services Computing (SCC), NY, USA (2015)
20. Ludwig, H., Keller, A.: Web Service Level Agreement (WSLA) Language Specification, pp. 1–110 (2003)
21. ISO/IEC: ISO/IEC 25010 Systems and Software Quality Requirements and Evaluation (SQuaRE)—System and software quality models (2011)
22. Lehmann, G., Blumendorf, M., Trollmann, F., Albayrak, S.: Meta-modeling runtime models. In: International Conference on Models in Software Engineering, pp. 209–223. Springer, Berlin (2010)
23. García, F., Bertoa, M.F., Calero, C., Vallecillo, A., Ruíz, F., Piattini, M., Genero, M.: Towards a consistent terminology for software measurement (2006)
24. Runeson, P., Höst, M.: Guidelines for conducting and reporting case study research in software engineering. Empirical Softw. Eng. **14**, 131–164 (2009)
25. Lethbridge, T.C., Sim, S.E., Singer, J.: Studying software engineers: data collection techniques for software field studies. Empirical Softw. Eng. **10**, 311–341 (2005)
26. Herold, S., Klus, H., Welsch, Y., Deiters, C., Rausch, A., Reussner, R., Krogmann, K., Koziolek, H., Mirandola, R., Hummel, B., Meisinger, M., Pfaller, C.: CoCoMe—the common component modeling example. Presented at the (2008)
27. Wieder, P., Butler, J.M., Theilmann, W., Yahyapour, R. (eds.): SLAs for Cloud Computing. Springer, New York (2011)
28. Quality Excellence for Suppliers of Telecommunications Forum (Quest Forum), TL 9000 Quality Management System Measurements Handbook 5.0 (2012)
29. Bauer, E., Adams, R.: Service Quality of Cloud-Based Applications. Wiley, Hoboken (2013)
30. Fernandez, A., Abrahão, S., Insfran, E.: A web usability evaluation process for model-driven web development. In: International Conference on Advanced Information Systems Engineering, pp. 108–122 (2011)

# A Motivation-Oriented Architecture Modelling for e-Healthcare Prosumption

Malgorzata Pankowska

**Abstract** The enterprise architecture (EA) is a coherent and consistent set of principles and rules that guide system design. Enterprise architecture is considered as strategic information assets, which determine the business mission and the business processes, in which the Information Communication Technologies (ICTs) are implemented. The EA acts as a basis to communicate the system knowledge to its stakeholders. In this paper, stakeholders' roles are emphasized as well as the motivation orientation in the enterprise architecture development is discussed. The following questions are formulated: who is the stakeholder of the EA, who is accountable and responsible for EA development, and what goals, constraints, and values are realized in the stakeholder activities' processes for the organization mission and vision by example of e-healthcare prosumption system.

**Keywords** Enterprise architecture · Stakeholders · Motivation · ArchiMate · e-healthcare · Prosumption

## 1 Introduction

Almost each business organization involves customers, suppliers, communities, employees, and experts, ICT people, financiers, media, and public administration institutions. They are mutually affected by the actions, decisions, policies and practices of the business firm as well as in the enterprise architecture development. The ISO/IEC 42010: 2007 shows that an architecture is the fundamental organization of a system, embodied in its components, their relationships to each other and the environment, and the principles governing its design and evolution. The goal of

---

A prior version of this paper has been published in the ISD2015 Proceedings (http://aisel.aisnet.org/isd2014/proceedings2015/).

---

M. Pankowska (✉)
University of Economics in Katowice, Katowice, Poland
e-mail: pank@ue.katowice.pl

D. Vogel et al. (eds.), *Transforming Healthcare Through Information Systems*,
Lecture Notes in Information Systems and Organisation 17,
DOI 10.1007/978-3-319-30133-4_3

EA is to create a unified ICT environment across the firm or all of the firm's business units with links to the business side of the organization, to promote alignment, standardization, reuse of existing ICT assets, and the sharing of common methods for project management and software development across the organization. The EA provides a holistic expression of the enterprise's strategies and their impact on business functions and processes, taking the firm's sourcing goals into consideration.

The paper aims to emphasize EA stakeholders' activities, their motivations, goals, constraints and values. The first part of the paper covers discussion on stakeholders' positions in the EA frameworks and models. The second part is to provide the present characteristics of e-healthcare prosumption. In the third part, the stakeholders' roles and motivations are formulated by example of e-healthcare prosumption architecture model.

## 2   Enterprise Architecture Framework Analysis

In this paper, the EA is considered as a bridge between strategy and design to develop business organization and to forecast its behaviour under specific conditions resulting from ICT implementation. There are many frameworks that support EA modelling and development:

- commercial frameworks: Zachman Framework (ZF); Architecture of Integrated Information Systems (ARIS); the Gartner Enterprise Architecture Framework (GEAF);
- defence industry frameworks: Command, Control, Communications, Computers, Intelligence, Surveillance, and Reconnaissance (C4ISR); UK Ministry of Defence Architecture Framework (MODAF);
- government frameworks: Federal Enterprise Architecture Framework (FEAF); Treasury Enterprise Architecture Framework (TEAF);
- enterprise developed frameworks: The Open Group Architecture Framework (TOGAF); Generalised Enterprise Reference Architecture and Methodology (GERAM); Computer Integrated Manufacturing Open System Architecture (CIMOSA);
- other frameworks: Compaq Services Architecture Methodology (CSAM); Dynamic Architecture (DYA); Systemic Enterprise Architecture Methodology (SEAM).

Only some of the above mentioned frameworks emphasize stakeholders' roles. The ZF provides a basic structure for organizing business architecture through dimensions such as data, function, network, people, time and motivation [1]. Zachman describes the ontology for the creation of EA through negotiations among several actors. The ZF presents various views and aspects of the EA in a highly structured and clear-cut form. It differentiates between the levels: Scope (contextual, planner view), Enterprise Model (conceptual, owner view), System Model (logical, designer view), Technology Model (physical, builder model), Detailed Representation (out-of-context, subcontractor), and Functioning Enterprise (user

**Table 1** The Zachman enterprise architecture framework

| | DATA What? | FUNCTION How? | NETWORK Where? | PEOPLE Who? | TIME When? | MOTIVATION Why? |
|---|---|---|---|---|---|---|
| SCOPE planner | Business things | Business processes | Locations | Business units | Events/cycles | Business strategies |
| ENTERPRISE owner | Semantic model | Business process model | Business logistics | Work flow model | Master schedule | Business plan |
| SYSTEM designer | Logical data model | Application architecture | Distributed system | Human interface | Processing structure | Business rules |
| TECHNOLOGY builder | Physical data model | System design | Technology architecture | Presentation architecture | Control structure | Rule design |
| OUT-OF-CONTEXT Subcontractor | Data definition | Program | Network architecture | Security architecture | Timing definition | Rule specification |
| ENTERPRISE User | Data | Function | Network | Organization | Schedule | Strategy |

*Source* [2]

view). Each of these views is presented as a row in the matrix (Table 1). The lower the row, the greater the degree of detail of the level represented. The model works with six aspects of the EA: Data (what), Function (how), Network (where), People (who), Time (when), Motivation (why). Each view (i.e., column) interrogates the architecture from a particular perspective. Taken together, all the views create a complete picture of the enterprise.

The Federal Enterprise Architecture Framework (FEAF) promotes interoperability and information sharing among USA governmental agencies [3]. The FEAF components of the enterprise architecture are as follows: architecture drivers, strategic direction, current architecture, target architecture, transitional processes, architectural segments, architectural models, and standards (Table 2).

The FEAF is to support establishing the scope of the enterprise architecture similarly as it is in the Zachman Framework. The FEAF method also accepts the actor-oriented approach, including Planner, Owner, Designer, Builder, and Subcontractor Perspective and demanding analysis of Data, Application and Technology Architecture from that five viewpoints. So, the holistic model of EA is the result of negotiations and compromises among different stakeholders.

The Treasury Enterprise Architecture Framework (TEAF) provides guidance and template for development and evolution of information systems architecture. The TEAF's functional, information and organizational architecture views allow for modelling the organization's processes and business operations. The enterprise architecture description is a matrix, with columns being views (functional, information, organizational and infrastructure) and rows being perspectives (planner, owner, designer, and builder). The matrix supports the realization of the transition strategy to new environment and establishing sustainability of the enterprise and its architecture [5].

The Compaq Services Architecture Methodology (CSAM) is a methodology complementary to Zachman's approach as it focuses on design decisions and not only on describing what exists on each level. The key issue is an understanding of the needs of all involved stakeholders. The CSAM method recommends using

**Table 2** The Federal Enterprise Architecture Framework

|  | Data architecture | Application architecture | Technology architecture |
|---|---|---|---|
| Planner perspective | List of business objects | List of business processes | List of business locations |
| Owner perspective | Semantic model | Business process model | Business logistics system |
| Designer perspective | Logical data model | Application architecture | System geographic deployment architecture |
| Builder perspective | Physical data model | Systems design | Technology architecture |
| Subcontractor perspective | Data dictionary | Programs | Network architecture |

*Source* [4]

different discipline-specific theories (e.g., Porter's value chain approach) for consideration of web of goals, principles, and obstacles [6].

In TOGAF approach, the stakeholders are people who have key roles in, or concerns about the system, for example as users, developers, or managers [7]. Different stakeholders with different roles in the system will have different concerns. Stakeholders can be individuals, teams or organizations. Concerns are the key interests that are crucially important to the stakeholders in the system, and determine the acceptability of the system. The problems of stakeholders are widely analysed in TOGAF modelling methodology. The Business Architecture Views address the concerns of users, planners, and business managers, and focus on the functional aspects of the system from the perspective of users of the system. The People view focuses on the human resource aspects of the system. The Business Process view deals with the user processes involved in the system. And the Business Function View deals with the functions required to support the processes.

Assuming that EA is the practice of describing the change of socio-technical organizations, their internal relationships and to the environment, the languages should be provided. The architecture description language is grounded in a domain and is associated to a context, as well as to other EA description languages. The languages are developed on many levels of abstractions. They concern both functional and non-functional EA aspects, and they are used to justify the EA concepts, and to recommend the proposed ICT projects [8]. They enable the general visualization of EA, a generic description, as well as look into particular detail, which is realized in the EA model. The frequently applied languages are as follows:

- Integrated Computer-Aided manufacturing (ICAM) DEFinition (IDEF) family of languages used to perform enterprise modelling and analysis (www.idef.com); their scope covers functional, process and data modelling, however there are no communication mechanisms between models and no motivation of EA considerations;
- Business Process Modelling Notation (BPMN) for business process modelling, therefore applications, motivations, or infrastructure are not covered by the language; BPMN aims at linking business process model design and process implementation. It is understandable by business analysts as well as technical developers;
- Testbed business modelling language and method, focusing on actors, business processes and data objects handled by business processes;
- Architecture of Integrated Information Systems (ARIS) for enterprise modelling and for business processes and information systems design;
- Event-driven Process Chains (EPCs) presented as ordered graph of events and functions;
- Unified Modelling Language (UML) intended to be used by information system designers to describe the systems in terms of object-oriented systems; UML use case diagrams are to show a number of actors and their connections to use cases that the system offers. Actors represent roles instead of real people, organizations or systems;

- Enterprise Distributed Object Computing (EDOC) provides a business collaboration architecture, a technology-independent business component architecture, and concepts for describing business processes, applications and infrastructure [9];
- ArchiMate (www.archimate.org) for describing business processes, organizational structures, information flows, ICT systems, and technical infrastructure;

The primary focus of ArchiMate language is to support stakeholders to address concerns regarding their business and the ICT systems. The motivational aspects in ArchiMate language correspond to the "Why" column of the Zachman framework. The Motivation extension of ArchiMate language adds motivational concepts such as stakeholder, driver, assessment, goal, principle, constraint and requirement [10]. The motivational element is defined as an element that provides the context or reason behind the architecture of an enterprise. Stakeholders represent groups of people or organizations that influence, guide, or constrain the enterprise. A stakeholder's concern represents a key interest that is crucially important to certain stakeholders in a system and determines the acceptability of the system. A concern may pertain to any aspect of the system functioning, development, or operation, including considerations such as performance, reliability, security, distribution and evolvability. Drivers represent internal or external factors which influence the plans and aims of an enterprise. An understanding of strengths, weaknesses, opportunities, and threats in relation to these drivers is necessary for the plans development. An example of an external drive is a change in regulation or compliance rules, which require change in the way an organization works, e.g., Sarbanes-Oxley in the US. An assessment represents the outcome of the analysis of some problems. The assessment is a stimulant of a change to the enterprise architecture, which is addressed by defining new business goals. A goal represents some effects that a stakeholder wants to achieve. It is a high level statement of intent or direction for an organization typically used to measure its success. The measure is an indicator or factor that can be tracked, usually on an ongoing basis, to determine success or alignment with objectives and goals. Principle is a qualitative statement of intent that should be met by the architecture. Requirement is also a qualitative statement, but of a business need that must be met by a particular architecture or work package. A work package is identified with a set of actions distinguished to achieve one or more objectives for the business. A work package can be a part of a project, a complete project or a program. Constraint is understood as an external factor that prevents an organization from pursuing particular approaches to meet its goal. Vicente et al., applied the ArchiMate language to manage a business plan for ICT management in an organized manner and according to ITIL guidelines [11].

ArchiMate is partly based on the ANSI/IEEE 1471-2000, Recommended Practice for Architecture Description of Software Intensive Systems. ArchiMate version 1.0 was formally approved as technical standard by the Board of The Open Group [12]. It should be noticed that ArchiMate is not designed to model the strategic, business network, financial or performance aspects of an enterprise. It focuses on the modelling of three layers, i.e., the business layer, the application layer, and the technology layer. The ArchiMate basic concepts are ambiguous and not easy to apply as intended. The language provides a means to extend the core set of concepts that are tailored towards such specific domains or applications [13]. Generally, the EA description languages are full of weaknesses, e.g.:

- the relations between domains are not well defined, and the models created on different levels are not fully integrated;
- the languages have a weak formal basis and lack of completely defined semantics;
- the languages lack the overall architectural vision and they are oriented towards specific domains;
- symbolic models express properties of architecture of systems. The models contain symbols that refer to reality.

## 3  e-Healthcare Prosumption

From patients' perspective, culture is a powerful force that shapes their motivations, lifestyles and healthcare service choices, therefore the e-healthcare prosumption is strongly based on local traditions. When developing international websites, e-healthcare institutions can achieve significant gains and cost reductions if they are able to centralize important care processes. A centralized global content management system enables e-healthcare knowledge provider to create, manage, publish and archive information in various formats and languages for use in many countries. Beyond that, a centralized system and workflows automate collaboration between important stakeholders in the web globalization process, such as project managers, translators, reviewers, experts, knowledge brokers and patients' guardians. A centralized web globalization team can be empowered (i.e., legitimated), responsible and accountable for the seamless integration of the web globalization workflows and coordination with regional and local communities. The centralized team could be needed to serve local teams in support of healthcare terminology management, healthcare evidence management, submitted information monitoring, intellectual property rights controlling, trainings, tools sharing, technology provision and maintenance, and quality assurance.

The basic premises of e-healthcare prosumption cover the development of technology supporting care at home, usage of in-house monitoring devices, enhancement of self-care for chronic disease management and post-acute monitoring. However, technology alone is not the key issue. Therefore, ICT must be incorporated into care management program personalized to an individual's needs. The patient-physician relationship system with more virtual interactions is needed to better coordinate care. e-Healthcare prosumption is identified with healthcare self-serviceability of Internet users, i.e., patients and their assistants, in a manner that empowers them to independently meet their own needs. Therefore, there is a need of an architectural framework that establishes that ICT must be engaged for a service, and concerns data analysis, data sourcing, data cleansing, and data integration.

Generally, healthcare is an extremely important, but complex and costly activity, because of its telemedicine infrastructure, and the human and physical resources it requires. These costs are continually increasing as public expectations for health-care rise, diseases such as cancer and mental illnesses are more prevalent, and demographics shift towards an aging population which require on average more frequent and longer periods of care [14]. The integration of digital information and exploitation of new technologies are having a significant impact on healthcare delivery and improving quality of life, while minimizing costs of the service. Many people prefer to discuss their problems with online advisors rather than immediately calling out their local doctor. Self-diagnosis has changed and recent advances in technology have enabled a vast range of more high-tech and affordable self-diagnosis tests to be available on the Internet as well as a huge number of more closely regulated products from street pharmacists. Internet pharmacies are gaining online, but some of their remedies may cause side effects, so self-medication can have serious consequences.

However, the potential benefits of e-healthcare prosumption are as follows:

- less face-to-face (F2F) contacts with physicians;
- a general culture shift to interact more through technology and new media;
- reduced waiting time because patients are not coming in as often;
- early avoidance of medical problems as self-diagnosis and self-testing are quicker;
- enabling the social networking to support assistance for surviving;
- reaching a wider geographically dispersed group that may not be able to, or want to meet physicians F2F.

e-Healthcare prosumption system should include questions and answers (Q&A) with medical professionals, as well as patient-to-patient communication. Moderation of social networking is important to ensure appropriate content and safeguarding vulnerable people. Therefore, e-healthcare prosumption system should cover two complementary subsystems:

- patient interactions and online experiences sharing under control of authority, i.e., knowledge brokers;
- offering clinical support in terms of Q&A sessions with health professionals and access to information resources.

There are some risks connected with the e-healthcare prosumption system:

- elaboration of the system content requires heavy input of medical knowledge;
- online safety and protection of website knowledge against destruction;
- losing contact with people who might be vulnerable, but will not ask for help;
- limited access to the mobile devices i.e., smartphones, wearable sensors;
- inappropriateness of the e-healthcare system for people with learning difficulties, brain tumours, memory problems or who are vulnerable;
- time required for development and verification of content for the forums is sometimes too long.

In the healthcare sector, knowledge brokering has been increasingly analyzed, because of the social needs to enhance the performance of health policies and care. Knowledge brokering process covers recognition, acquisition, assimilation, transformation and exploitation or application of new knowledge [15]. Knowledge brokering has been recently enhanced through the use of Web platforms, i.e., websites, Facebook, blogs, Twitter, newsletters, wikis, YouTube, LinkedIn, podcasts, chatting, RSS feeds. In social networks, a knowledge broker could be responsible for mobilization of the stakeholders interested in the knowledge production and the use of knowledge.

In the aspect of validity, the patients and their guardians need the computerized access to three types of knowledge:

- knowledge concerning incidents and problems, which are the results of insufficient learning or weaknesses of e-healthcare application. The problems MUST BE solved by medicine experts;
- questions, which answers are delivered by an expert or possibly by a user with the help of experts. The answers of the questions SHOULD BE received and the further works on e-healthcare system development and extension are necessary;
- suggestions provided by users as the result of their own experiences, wisdom and practices. Suggestions COULD BE further surveyed, analysed and discussed with a body of experts, presented in the form of case studies, and explained for the end user.

In the aspect of knowledge source, the e-healthcare knowledge can be differentiated between knowledge about the patients, knowledge from the patients, and knowledge for the patient. Knowledge about the patient comprises information about socio-demographic characteristics, their habits, health status, style of life and work, personal needs, abilities and illnesses as the results of analyses, interviews and observations. Knowledge from the patient mostly arrives in a direct way. The patient informs the physician about his health problems, illnesses and delivers basic health status parameters, e.g. blood pressure. That knowledge is gathered in diagnosis process through testing and self-testing, hospital and home monitoring or self-monitoring. When the patient shares his knowledge with another patient or physician, the latter is able to identify a possible knowledge gap and to further develop patient's knowledge to fulfil the "non-knowledge" space. The knowledge for the patients encourages them to self-monitor and recuperate.

# 4 Stakeholder Emphasis in e-Healthcare Prosumption Architecture Modelling

Stakeholders are groups and individuals who have a stake in the success or failure of a business. They are people for whom the value is created, who are beneficiaries of the EA development decision, and whose rights are enabled.

For e-healthcare system development, the following stakeholders have been specified:

- stakeholders, whose concerns address the consistency of the overall architecture of e-healthcare prosumption system or the strategic direction to follow in accordance with the political goals of e-healthcare prosumption, i.e., governmental agencies, healthcare associations, which accomplish these goals through the delivery of educational programs and knowledge for patients in a partnership with other health related organizations, academic institutions, government, technology community and standards bodies;
- stakeholders, who are the recipients of knowledge provided for patients in the knowledge supply process in the e-healthcare prosumption system. Basically, they are patients, their family members, health care assistants, friends, physicians and other healthcare personnel, or even anonymous Internet reviewers;
- stakeholders, who are involved during an ICT project to build or change a system, these are the project sponsors, the solution architects, knowledge brokers, healthcare process analysts, and project leaders;
- stakeholders that are charged with strategic planning, decision making, e.g., Chief Information Officer (CIO), Chief Security Officer (CSO), medical experts, knowledge engineers;
- stakeholders that are responsible for the controlling of how efficiently ICT is used in an enterprise. This is typically an internal or external auditor.

Stakeholders of the e-healthcare prosumption system contribute to the three kinds of architecture (i.e., Business, Application and Technology Infrastructure) in one consistent way. An end user may want to change the information requirement, if technology (i.e., wearable monitoring devices) does not constrain what can be achieved, or an architect may need to reconsider a design if new non-functional requirements arise. Architects in each of the architectural areas also influence each other's decisions. Software architects designing for software reliability need the design support of system architects as well as of knowledge brokers and end users. The knowledge based e-healthcare prosumption system development relies not only on system developer research aims and epistemological stance, but also on organizational, historical, cultural evidence and personal factors, which are not problems to be solved, but factors that must be included in practical research design.

For e-healthcare prosumption architecture modelling, the ArchiMate language is applied to emphasize the stakeholders in a suitable manner to support business agility (see Fig. 1).

A system architecture model in ArchiMate is organized into some basic layers:

- BUSINESS containing following elements: actor (i.e., Patient), role (i.e., e-Healthcare Service Prosumer, Knowledge Broker), process (i.e., e-Healthcare Consultation Process covering 17 subprocesses), service (i.e., e-healthcare Service Information Browsing, e-Healthcare Service Conceptualization, e-Healthcare Service Knowledge Component Registration, e-Healthcare Service Knowledge Components' Catalogue, e-Healthcare Service Knowledge

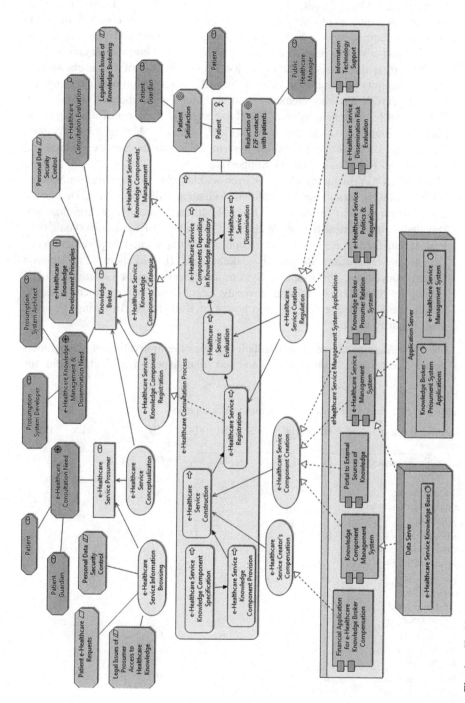

**Fig. 1** e-Healthcare prosumption architecture model

Components' Management). In the paper, the e-healthcare knowledge management is component-oriented. Therefore, each service consists of some knowledge components, which are designed, constructed and selected to provide optimal advice to patients and their guardians. The knowledge components can be further designed as learning objects for education of end users and for their community considered as organization of learning good medical practices.

- APPLICATION covering elements such as Financial Application, Knowledge Component Management System, Portal to External Sources of Knowledge (e.g. libraries, journals, document repositories), Service Management System, Knowledge Broker-Patient Relation System, e-Healthcare Service Politics and Regulations, Risk Evaluation, IT Support.
- TECHNOLOGY including elements such as Data Server, Application Server.
- MOTIVATION containing the following elements: drivers (i.e., e-Healthcare Consultation Needs), principles (i.e., e-Healthcare Knowledge Development Principles), assessment (i.e., e-Healthcare Consultation Evaluation), goals (i.e., Patient Satisfaction, Reduction of F2F contacts with patients), requirements (i.e., Patient e-e-Healthcare Requests), stakeholders (i.e., Patient, Prosumption System Developer, Prosumption System Architect, Patient Guardian, Public Healthcare Manager), constraints covering Legal Issues of Prosumer Access to Healthcare Knowledge, Legalization Issues of Knowledge Brokering, Personal Data Security Control.

The ArchiMate as a modelling standard explains the motivation of stakeholders to develop enterprise architecture. Later on that aspect was included in the

**Table 3** RACI chart for e-healthcare prosumption stakeholders

| Key management practices | PG | HA | MS | II | SG | KB | ISD | ITA | PHM |
|---|---|---|---|---|---|---|---|---|---|
| e-Healthcare strategic planning | I | C | C | R | A | C | R | R | C |
| Understanding e-healthcare knowledge brokering | C | C | C | R | C | A | R | R | C |
| e-Healthcare prosumption vision development | R | A | C | C | C | R | I | I | C |
| The cultural environment capabilities and performance | A | A | R | R | C | R | R | A | C |
| The target IT capabilities development | C | C | C | R | A | C | A | A | C |
| The ICT investment development and project planning | R | R | R | A | A | R | R | C | C |

Enterprise Business Motivation Model (EBMM) that aims at illustrating how the actions of a company are aligned with its objectives [16].

Proposed in Table 3 e-healthcare prosumption organizational structure covers the most important stakeholders, i.e., Patients and their Guardians (PG), Healthcare Associations (HA), Medical Staff (MS), Institutional Investors (II), State Government (SG), Knowledge Brokers (KB), Information Systems Developers (ISD), Information Communication Technology Architects (ICTA), Public Healthcare Managers (PHM). Their activities are further precisely specified and verified in particular projects.

It should be noticed that particularly important role of e-healthcare prosumption development belongs to governmental agencies, healthcare associations, and ICT Architects to ensure that prosumption systems will be developed under control of professionals. End users, i.e., e-healthcare prosumers, patients and their guardians (PG) will be the most important beneficiaries of the system and the recipients of distributed knowledge. The quality of e-healthcare knowledge provided online should be ensured and verified by knowledge brokers (KB), information systems developers (ISD), ICT architects (ICTA), and medical staff (MS), however, the consultative roles of prosumers cannot be excluded.

The e-healthcare prosumption system stakeholders realize activities, which can be integrated and consolidated in the RACI model. The "RACI" acronym is developed as follows:

- RESPONSIBLE: refers to the person who must ensure that activities are completed successfully;
- ACCOUNTABLE: refers to the person or group, who has the authority to approve or accept the execution of an activity;
- CONSULTED: refers to the people whose opinions are sought on an activity (two-way communication);
- INFORMED: refers to the people who are kept up to date on the progress of an activity (one-way communication) [17].

ArchiMate as an architecture modelling tool seems to be appropriate for the visualization of EA stakeholders. Other architecture modelling tools, e.g., Enterprise Architecture Modelio focus on information modelling and specification of an enterprise ontology. They are suitable for applications and system design in UML and BPMN languages. The ArchiMate Canvas Model allows to catch intangible requirements and emphasize the stakeholders' place in the system architecture (Fig. 2). Presented in Fig. 2 e-Healthcare Prosumption Architecture Canvas Model includes specified: Key Partnerships, Key Activities, Key Resources, Value Propositions, Customer Relationships, Customer Segments, Channels for Communication, Cost Structure, and Revenue Streams. This specification allows to consider e-Healthcare Prosumption System as a project, or a program. Studying the Canvas Model enables analysing the most important functionalities and non-functional requirements of the proposed system architecture. The Canvas Model permits for consideration of the stakeholder relationships, however the

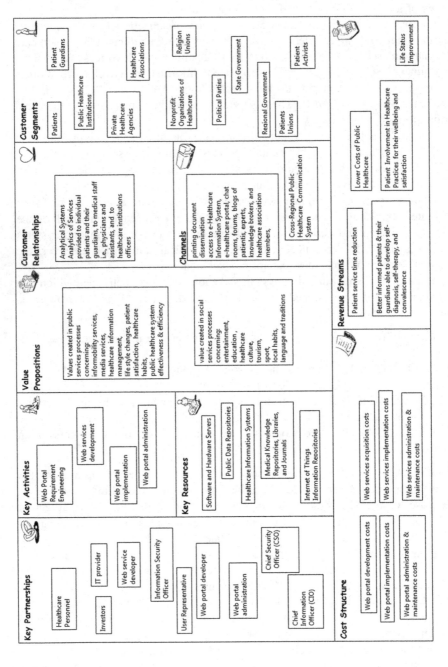

**Fig. 2** e-Healthcare prosumption architecture canvas model

motivations of their behaviour are not clearly visible in ArchiMate diagrams. The determined list of value propositions can be identified with the list of concerns for the EA motivation modelling and analyses.

## 5 Conclusions

The development of stakeholder oriented architecture framework and methodology is still a challenge. Some good works have been done by the Open Group, therefore the e-healthcare prosumption architecture model was done in ArchiMate language. The proposed architecture model is developed to emphasize the stakeholder position as well as an important proposal that could be further realized. The EA stakeholders are individuals, groups, or organizations who may affect, be affected by, or perceive themselves to be affected by a decision, activity, or outcome of a project. Within the community of stakeholders for e-healthcare prosumption system architecture development a particularly important role belongs to the knowledge brokers. Further research works should focus on designing tasks for them as well as on the development of learning objects for healthcare knowledge management.

## References

1. Zachman, J.A.: Frameworks standards: what's it all about? In: Kappelman, L.A. (ed.) The SIM Guide to Enterprise Architecture, pp. 66–70. CRC Press, Boca Raton (2010)
2. Minoli, D.: Enterprise Architecture A to Z, Frameworks, Business Process Modeling, SOA, and Infrastructure Technology. CRC Press, London (2008)
3. A Practical Guide to Federal Enterprise Architecture, version 1.0., General Accounting Office, Office of Management and Budget. Access March 2012, http://www.gao.gov/bestpractices/bpeaguide.pdf (2001)
4. Federal Enterprise Architecture Framework, version 1.1. CIO Council, Access May 2012, http://www.cio.gov/documents/fedarch1.pdf (1999)
5. Bernus, P., Nemes, L., Schmidt, G.: Handbook on Enterprise Architecture. Springer, Berlin (2003)
6. Compaq Services Architecture Methodology (CSAM). Access April 2015, http://www.compaq.com/services/ (2002)
7. Desfray, P., Raymond, G.: Modeling Enterprise Architecture with TOGAF. Morgan Kaufmann Waltham, Elsevier, Amsterdam (2014)
8. Kotze, P., Tsogang, M., van der Merwe, A.: A framework for creating pattern languages for enterprise architecture. In: Aier, S., Ekstedt, M., Matthes, F., Proper, E., Sanz, J.L. (eds.) Trends in Enterprise Architecture Research and Practice-Driven Research on Enterprise Transformation, Lecture Notes in Business Information Processing, pp. 1–20. Springer, Berlin (2012)
9. Lankhorst, M.: Enterprise Architecture at Work. Springer, Heidelberg (2013)
10. Engelsman, W., Jonkers, H., Quartel, D.: Supporting Requirements Management in TOGAF and ArchiMate. Access March 2015 http://www.opengroup.org (2010)
11. Vicente, M., Gama, N., Mira de Silva, M.: Modeling ITIL business motivation model in ArchiMate. In: Falcao e Cunha, J., Snene, M., Novoa, H. (eds.) Exploring Services Sciences, pp. 86–99. Springer, Berlin (2013)

12. Glissmann, S., Sanz, J.: Business architectures for the design of enterprise service systems. In: Maglio, P.P., Kieliszewski, Ch.A., Spohrer, J.C. (eds.) Handbook of Service Science, Service Science: Research and Innovations in the Service Economy, pp. 251–283. Springer, Heidelberg (2010)
13. Jonkers, H., Groenewegen, L., Bonsangue, M., van Buuren R.: A language for enterprise modelling. In: Lankhorst, M. (ed.) Enterprise Architecture at Work, pp. 85–118. Springer, Berlin (2009)
14. Adams, A.A., McCrindle, R.J.: Pandora's Box, Social and Professional Issues of the Information Age. Wiley, Chichester (2008)
15. Lamari, M., Ziam, S.: Profile of knowledge brokering in the Web 2.0 era. In: International Conference on Information Society (i-Society 2014), pp. 345–355 (2004)
16. Malik, A.N.: Enterprise Business Motivation Model, Full Model Documentation. Access October 2015, http://motivationmodel.com/download/EBMM%20Report%20v42.pdf (2014)
17. Certificate of Governance of Information Technology CGEIT Review Manual 2015, ISACA, Rolling Meadows (2014)

# A Proposed Framework for Examining Information Systems Security Research: A Multilevel Perspective

Ruilin Zhu and Lech Janczewski

**Abstract** As information security becomes increasingly important, more research is being conducted in this area. In an attempt to better understand current research activities in Information Systems Security (ISsec) and to guide future explorations, a number of authors have made tentative attempts to survey/review the existing literature. However the criteria employed in these reviews are neither consistent nor complete which weakens their validity. Drawing on previous research and Multilevel Theory, we propose an improved examination framework for systematically investigating ISsec research. This framework will allow researchers to gain a more thorough understanding of what has been done so far and to target future research efforts more effectively.

**Keywords** Information systems security · Examining framework · Paradigm · Theory · Method · Analysis

## 1 Introduction

The last few decades have witnessed the widespread adoption and development of Information Systems (IS) to the point where they are now deployed in almost every organization. Organizations of all kinds and sizes have adopted IS for administrative, managerial, marketing, communication and production purposes in an effort to adapt to a fast-changing world and enhance competitiveness. The wide use of IS has sparked a series of research activities in this area that aim at boosting efficiency

---

A prior version of this paper has been published in the ISD2015 Proceedings (http://aisel.aisnet.org/isd2014/proceedings2015/).

---

R. Zhu (✉) · L. Janczewski
The University of Auckland, Auckland, New Zealand
e-mail: ruilin.zhu@auckland.ac.nz

L. Janczewski
e-mail: l.janczewski@auckland.ac.nz

© Springer International Publishing Switzerland 2016
D. Vogel et al. (eds.), *Transforming Healthcare Through Information Systems*,
Lecture Notes in Information Systems and Organisation 17,
DOI 10.1007/978-3-319-30133-4_4

49

and reliability. Methodology in this research area is continuously evolving, and this has had a clear and direct influence on the development of IS itself [1].

Information Systems security (ISsec), however, has received little attention compared to other IS issues [2]. According to a survey released by the UK's Department for Business, Innovation and Skills in 2013, 42 % of large organizations do not provide any ongoing security awareness training to their staff, despite the fact that 78 % of these organizations had been attacked by an unauthorized outsider in the previous year [3]. But safe, robust and reliable IS are crucial if an organization is to achieve its business goals [4].

The need to develop effective ISsec should be driving academic activity, but published anecdotal evidence and existing ISsec survey research suggest that research in ISsec lags behind the general advance in IS [5], and that it is often perceived as esoteric and inconclusive. The few existing studies are isolated rather than systematic, and ISsec research generally has been disjointed. Those studies that do contain in-depth analysis only concentrate on a small number of ISsec research outputs, while those that examine a large number of articles merely focus on certain criteria rather than taking an overall view. Thus, a comprehensive study of ISsec research is overdue.

The main purpose of this research, therefore, is to provide practical suggestions to refine the existing examining framework which will allow researchers to conduct in-depth, systematic reviews/surveys of existing material, thereby facilitating reflection upon previous ISsec research and supporting future study.

We aim to briefly describe previous reviews of ISsec research, to analyse the criteria employed in this research and to offer suggestions for future activities. Thus, Sect. 2 presents an overview of previous research efforts and the criteria they have adopted, Sect. 3 details the Multilevel Theory for the examining framework, and Sect. 4 considers the components that should be taken into account in the examining framework. We set out a plan for future study in Sect. 5, while Sect. 6 concludes the research by summarizing our findings.

## 2 Related Work

Mounting threats to IS security and the growing attention being paid to this issue have prompted a range of studies on ISsec. However, although a number of important threads have been developed in ISsec research, these threads have not been woven together into a cohesive fabric. To achieve a better understanding of current ISsec research activities, and to establish a clear research pattern, a number of authors have attempted to examine ISsec research.

Baskerville [6] pioneered exploration into ISsec research by detailing the mismatch between system development methods in general and security development methods in particular. He suggested that to survey and compare security analysis and design methods, their general characteristics are needed. The taxonomy, simple but useful, relates the evolution of information systems security methods to the perspective of the broader information systems development community, and thus is chosen as the criterion.

The study of ISsec research as a discipline in its own right did not emerge until the 2000s. Dhillon and Backhouse [7] analysed eleven ISsec studies by adopting sociological paradigms developed by Burrell and Morgan [8] to illustrate the need for understanding the social as well as the technical aspects of ISsec. They posited that while IS research in general had moved away from a narrow technical viewpoint, ISsec research was still dominated by technical and functionalist preconceptions, and that the use of socio-organizational perspectives to understand ISsec was still at the theory-building stage.

Villarroel et al. [9] critically reviewed eleven secure system design methodologies, paying particular attention to their technological and practical implications. Others [5, 10] went further, undertaking relatively comprehensive comparisons of methodologies. These later studies were the first to adopt systematic criteria (i.e. theory, method, and topic) to review existing research.

Although these studies cast some light on ISsec research, they are not without their limitations. Baskerville's [6] research was conducted in the early days of IS, before the development of appropriate research mechanisms and standards, while Villarroel et al. [9] concentrated only on the development of secure IS and system design methods and methodologies, which is only one of the three research tracks within the ISsec field. Furthermore, they listed but did not explain their chosen criteria.

Although Dhillon and Backhouse [7] tried to deepen the discussion, their arguments were not based on widely accepted theoretical paradigms and were bounded with the concept of development of secure IS, which weakens their applicability. Moreover, they adopted sociological theory but ignored the key influence of IS theoretical paradigms on ISsec research. Finally, they reviewed a limited number of articles which raises questions about the generalizability of their criteria.

The research of Siponen et al. [5] was relatively systematic in that their choice of theory, method and topic as the three examining factors was consistent with the Reticulated Model of Science [11]. However, separating these factors out in this way is inconsistent with the integrated nature of the research process, and this set of criteria neglect the analysis stage altogether. Siponen et al.'s most recent research [5] was conducted in 2008, but during the past few years, tremendous changes have taken place in ISsec and numerous advances have been made. Our research aims to reflect these changes and to incorporate more recent contributions.

In addition, previous ISsec research examining work has centred on comparing and constructing the theoretical paradigm, theory, and method, while often discounting or oversimplifying the context in which the ISsec phenomenon was embedded. This is to say that most frameworks do not take into account multiple levels of analysis, suggesting that they are no longer effective and efficient in determining the appropriateness and usefulness of relevant research.

In summary, previous ISsec studies have shortcomings which seriously impair their validity. In theoretical terms, they do not take the methodological perspective into consideration, meaning that their criteria are patchy and inconclusive. From a practical perspective, they neglect the role of research analysis and the way that ISsec phenomenon arose.

## 3  Theoretical Framework

Multilevel Theory (MT) has its first underpinning from General Systems Theory (GST), which was shaped and became the dominant perspective in the twentieth century. It originates from the notion of a holistic view—that the whole is greater than the sum of its parts. According to Klein and Kozlowski [12], the primary goal of GST is to establish general understanding across phenomena in order to generalize key principles.

In contrast, the Micro-Macro Perspective (MiMaP) recognises that while micro phenomena are embedded within a macro context, macro phenomena often emerges from micro elements [13]. The Micro Perspective emphasizes the variations among individuals that affect his/her behaviour and the Macro Perspective focuses on the collective response from a group of individuals regardless of individual variation.

MT, however, engenders a more integrated view towards organizational phenomenon by combining MiMaP. It spans the levels of organizational behaviours and performance and bridges the micro-macro divide. It acknowledges the influence of the organization on individuals' actions and the influence of individual's action on an organization thereby resulting in a richer and deeper understanding of the organizational phenomenon [14].

The central concept of MT is that it accepts the notion that an organizational phenomenon resides in nested arrangements. In this sense, the individual is nested in groups or other subunits, which are also nested in higher hierarchies of organizations and industry, the layers both in turn embedded in certain environments. Hitt et al. [13] point out that this nesting arrangement has certain implications for organizational related research despite the fact that the exact number and nature of layers vary depending on different situations.

MT brings at least two aspects of benefits to scholars [15, 16]. Firstly, MT connects the previously unlinked constructs within organizational literature so as to facilitate the synthesis within the research. Secondly, it illustrates the contexts surrounding individual variation and organizational aggregation respectively, which yields important and profound practical insights.

Rousseau [17] provided a useful set of guidance for undertaking MT-oriented research. She advised that scholars should simultaneously consider the levels of theory, measurement, and analysis for the constructs included in their investigations. Level of theory refers to the focal unit to which the investigations are meant to apply to. "Level of measurement refers to the unit to which the data are directly attached, and the level of analysis is the unit to which data are assigned for hypothesis testing and statistical analysis" [17]. As within the ISsec context, they signal the components of research theory, research method, and research analysis respectively, which will be discussed along with research paradigm in the next section.

# 4  A Proposed Examining Framework

The IS community's interest in methodological issues has grown considerably, as methodology is of great importance in directing research activities. These activities may include administering and analysing a survey, conducting controlled experiments, engaging in ethnography or participant observation, and developing root definitions and conceptual models. Research methodology may be described as a clearly defined sequence of operations [18, 19]. More generally, a methodology is a structured set of guidelines designed to assist the researcher in generating valid and reliable research results. This methodology will be built upon a set of assumptions, methods and techniques [20]. It is our view that the examining framework should reflect all these methodological components; in other words, it should encompass paradigm, theory, method and analysis. Moreover we contend that to fully understand the current ISsec research and to better direct future efforts, it is crucial to examine it in terms of how it unfolds the research analysis with its other parts, such as the research method, at each level or some levels—the particular focus/foci in the hierarchy at which the ISsec phenomenon was embedded. Accordingly, the following sections draw on existing research to discuss how these four components should be incorporated into the framework.

## 4.1  Research Paradigm

All IS scholars take on their research holding a number of explicit and implicit philosophical assumptions about the nature of human organizations, the nature of their particular search/review and the expected results. These assumptions play a crucial role in guiding the IS research procedure and directly affect the likelihood they will get a result, as well as the nature of these results; in other words, the assumptions that are adopted will determine the research approach and the potential research outcomes.

A number of theoretical perspectives have been employed in the IS domain. Orlikowski and Baroudi [21] were the first to identify the various paradigms employed in IS literature, which they did by surveying 155 research articles published between 1983 and 1988. Following Chua's classification of research epistemologies [22], Orlikowski and Baroudi identified the positivist, interpretive and critical paradigms as the most widely used. The positivist paradigm aims to test theory to arrive at a better predictive understanding of a phenomenon. The paradigm is premised on the assumption that the phenomenon can be understood by objectively measuring a set of known fixed variables. By contrast, the interpretive paradigm assumes that scholars are able to create their own subjective understanding by interacting with the world around them; phenomena are understood by accessing the meanings that are assigned to them. Finally, the critical paradigm critiques deep-rooted contradictions within social systems with the aim of emancipating individuals from restrictive social conditions.

| Table 1 Three types of research paradigm | Research paradigm | |
|---|---|---|
| | 1 | Positivist |
| | 2 | Interpretive |
| | 3 | Critical |

Since these three paradigms guide nearly all research in IS, they were adopted as the criterion for the philosophic assumption component (Table 1).

## 4.2 Research Theory

Theory, illustrating the scholars' cognitive aim and facilitating intervention and action, is generally developed to describe, explain and enhance our understanding of the world and to predict what will happen in the future. Numerous theories have been adopted in ISsec research; 38 were identified by Siponen et al. [5]. It would be inefficient, if not impossible, to develop a framework that statistically examines the theoretical perspective of every piece of ISsec research—in any case, such attention to detail may blur the overall picture. It is therefore necessary to choose an alternative theory-related criterion. This criterion must be easy to manipulate while accurately reflecting the range of theoretical perspectives employed.

Gregor [23] discerned five distinct theoretical approaches. Studies employing analysis theory, the most basic type, describe what has been found in previous research thereby classifying specific characteristics of research entity, such as individual, team or phenomenon. Studies employing explanation theory seek to explain how and why phenomena occur, while prediction theory's primary goal is to take these explanatory factors into account in order to make logical and testable predictions about the future. Studies combining explanation and prediction theory seek to demonstrate the existence of a phenomenon, how, why and when it occurs, and what will happen in the future. Finally, studies employing design and action theory seek to explain the principles by which systems are created and thus guide the development of IS.

This five-type typology of theory, indicating the cognitive aim where the research focuses, represents the theoretical foundation of IS and was therefore adopted as the criterion for categorizing theoretical approaches in ISsec research (Table 2).

| Table 2 Five types of research theory | Research theory | |
|---|---|---|
| | 1 | Analysis |
| | 2 | Explanation |
| | 3 | Prediction |
| | 4 | Explanation and prediction |
| | 5 | Design and action |

## 4.3   Research Method

Significant attention has been paid to the research methods that have been applied in IS research, as they reflect implicit or explicit assumptions on the part of the researcher about the nature of the world and of knowledge. The research method can be viewed as the operational dimension for provoking a response from the world. The nature of the response depends on both the world and the underlying assumptions. Different methods generate information about different aspects of the world. This information is used to construct theories about the world, which in turn condition our experience of the world.

It is commonly held that research methods are bound to particular paradigms and that as these paradigms are incommensurable, it is illogical to mix methods from different paradigms. However, Mingers [20] asserts that it is both desirable and feasible to combine different research methods to gain richer and more reliable research results.

In an effort to well situate the position of research methods and encourage the adoption of a wider range of methodological approaches, several authors have sought to classify existing studies by research method. This has been approached in various ways; Benbasat et al. [24], for example, compared studies employing qualitative research methods to those using experimental and survey-based research methods, while Alavi et al. [25] divided the empirical studies they looked at into eight categories according to whether they were based on laboratory experiments, field experiments, field studies, case studies, surveys, MIS instruments, ex-post descriptions or other methods. Similarly, Orlikowski and Baroudi [21] surveyed 155 articles, classifying studies according to whether they were based on surveys, laboratory experiments, case studies, mixed methods, instrument development, protocol analysis or action research.

Among these different taxonomies the most consistent comparisons are between empirical and non-empirical [25] and quantitative and qualitative [24] methods. However, both of these general classifications have limitations. Regarding the specific types of method taxonomy, it is again too detailed for researchers to see the whole picture. In fact, there are more than ten frequently used methods in current IS and most of them can be employed across the paradigms. With this classification, it is difficult to map out the general picture of the coherent research activities. As for the straightforward dichotomy of method taxonomy, in contrast, it is too simplistic for researchers to explore the in-depth implications stemming from the research activities. Klein and Myers [26] indicate that quantitative/qualitative research can be positivist, interpretive or critical. Moreover, some research methods can be used in the context of both quantitative and qualitative research. In other words, this classification is useful in understanding the research approaches that the researchers, but not efficient to determine the appropriateness of the paradigms and theories and the overall consistence of the whole research activities.

In this sense, method taxonomy should not only be concerned with method itself, but also with theoretical considerations—it needs to be abstract enough to

**Table 3** Two main types of research method

| Research method | | |
|---|---|---|
| 1 | Explanation paradigm (Behavioural paradigm) | Quantitative method |
| | | Qualitative method |
| 2 | Improvement paradigm | Design science method |

categorize a range of research but concrete enough to render rich implications to the research activities.

We chose the taxonomy of method proposed by von Alan et al. [27]. These authors group methods under the explanation (behavioural) paradigm and the improvement paradigm. The behavioural paradigm seeks to develop and verify theories that explain or predict human or organizational behaviour, while the design paradigm seeks to extend the boundaries of human and organizational capabilities by creating new and innovative artefacts. Both paradigms are fundamental to the IS discipline, positioned as it is at the confluence of people, organizations and technology. They signify the research operational dimensions where the research data is collected and attempts are made (Table 3).

## 4.4   Research Analysis

Analysis is an indispensable part of most IS research articles, as this is where the preliminary research results are positioned within a broader context. The analysis presents the research outcomes, summarising the outputs from theoretical exploration and connecting theory with practice by explaining how the research applies to a real social setting. The fact that this essential stage has always been ignored in previous reviews of ISsec research reduces the value of these reviews. In this research, we endeavour to incorporate this component into the examining framework.

In terms of the level of analysis, scholars have a long history of recognising that organizational phenomena unfold within complex and dynamic systems [28], yet their scholarship often neglects the multilevel dynamics of these social systems [29]. Adopting either a micro or a macro stance yields an incomplete understanding of behaviours occurring at either level [30], and a proliferation of diverse research paradigms [13]. Analysis enabled by MT is one of the ways to stimulate the development of a more expansive paradigm for an in-depth understanding of organizational phenomenon.

By definition, IS mainly deals with the relationship between information technology and organizations, and ISsec is no exception. By their very nature, organizations are multi-level as individuals work in groups, and teams within organizations that also interact with other organizations within society [15]. In addition, no construct is level free as it is tied to one or more organizational levels. Thus, to examine organizational phenomena is to encounter level issues.

In particular, multilevel thinking has surfaced from empirical endeavours aimed at understanding ISsec by examining organizational-level factors and individual behaviours. Most research explores security-related phenomenon by examining them at single level. For instance, the concept of security awareness arises from the process of technological advances, which are featured with three-stage development [31]. Siponen [32] introduced a five-dimension information security awareness framework, which tends to address the concern of organizational and societal level respectively. This has sparked a series of conceptual studies over the following periods. In particular, Puhakainen [33] proposed a design theory for improving information security awareness campaigns at group level while D'Arcy et al. [34] suggested that organizations can adopt user awareness of security policies as one of the three security countermeasures to reduce the information systems misuse at the organizational level.

As the field of ISsec thrives, however, researchers tend to develop a more complex understanding of the phenomenon from different levels. In the security awareness research stream, some scholars came to notice that the user dimension of the problem is nonetheless neglected [35]. As a complement, some scholars explored the relationship between awareness and behaviour. Albrechtsen and Hovden [36] specifically figured out the positive effect of awareness on behaviour. As a step further, Bulgurcu et al. [37] conducted an empirical exploration that analysed the roles of information security awareness on an employee's compliance behaviour. As a result, Tariq et al. [38] call for studies that examine the issue from an individual perspective.

The efforts above of examining the phenomenon from different perspectives and the trend of integrating focal levels suggest that organizational policy and individual behaviours both play important roles in security awareness. Thus, the explorations on security awareness is inherently a multilevel problem. Similar revelations could be drawn from other streams in ISsec, such as privacy and BYOD (Bring Your Own Device), etc.

Generally, by adopting MT, we argue that organizational outcomes of interest to ISsec scholars could be better understood if they break out of the level-specific mind-sets. In other words, a piece of ISsec research could be thoroughly examined by utilising MT-related elements. In addition, the adoption of level of analysis also necessities the consistence of examining efforts across the theory, method (measurement), and analysis.

Management research has generally adopted four levels of analysis—these have been adapted for ISsec research [39]. At the individual level, ISsec has been studied in terms of the factors that affect individuals, while at the level of groups/teams, ISsec has been studied in terms of the factors that foster or curb the security of a certain group. Research at the organizational level has focused on the impact technology and new products/business/structures have on various types of organization. Finally, research at the societal level has focused on the management of ISsec and the emergence of new threats (Table 4).

**Table 4** Four levels of research analysis

| Research analysis | |
| --- | --- |
| 1 | Individual level |
| 2 | Group/team level |
| 3 | Organizational level |
| 4 | Societal level |

## 4.5  Examining Framework

To sum up, the theoretical framework consists of four components: research paradigm, research theory, research method and research analysis with a concentration on Multilevel Theory. Together, these cover the whole research procedure and address the concerns from the theoretical, methodological, and practical perspectives (Table 5).

The advantages of this comprehensive framework for examining ISsec research are threefold. Firstly, distinct from the previous frameworks that either focused on certain component(s) of ISsec research or were based on some less accepted paradigms, our framework, adapted from widely-recognised and well-established research, takes into account all necessary components of the ISsec research activity. This is able to facilitate the possibility of obtaining a more thorough and profound understanding of the ISsec research by examining its integrated procedure with four objectives. Secondly, the previous studies that examined the theory and/or method predominately focused on the specific type of theory or method employed. One unavoidable problem stemming from that notion is that it is difficult if not impossible to work out the latent connection between a certain set of theory and

**Table 5** Framework for examining information systems security research

| Objective | Philosophical assumption | Cognitive aim | Operational dimension | Interpretive level |
| --- | --- | --- | --- | --- |
| Procedure | Research paradigm | Research theory (level of theory) | Research method (level of measurement) | Research analysis (level of analysis) |
| Criteria | Positivist | Analysis | Explanation/behavioural | Individual level |
| | Interpretive | Explanation | Improvement | Group/team level |
| | Critical | Prediction | | Organizational level |
| | | Explanation and prediction | | Societal level |
| | | Design and action | | |

method given the fact that there are at least dozens of different theories and methods. However, our framework is the first attempt, as far as we know, to map out an examining framework that closely combines each component by integrating their underlying assumptions, thereby enabling us to seek the possible relationship from a coherent and interconnected perspective. Thirdly this expanded examining framework is able to examine the ISsec research activities from a holistic and integrated perspective as it evaluates the research work from different levels that the concepts or constructs are nested on. The benefits it brings are evident: on the one hand, it fosters the synergy within ISsec by rendering a rich portrait of organizational phenomenon where the ISsec research have been unfurled, and on the other hand, it illuminates the steps that the ISsec research have taken or will take, individually, collectively, and progressively towards the organizational problems.

## 5   Limitations and Future Work

There are some limitations to the research at this stage. Firstly, there was only a limited number of reviews/surveys of ISsec research to draw on. Similarly, the fact that there are only a few typology studies on ISsec made the selection of criteria more difficult. Three of the four components (research paradigm being the exception) do not possess generally recognized typology, and potential criteria had to be selected from a comparatively small pool. Thirdly, the concept of level analysis has been borrowed from the discipline of management and adjusted to fit the context of ISsec. In addition, we have not yet conducted an empirical review/survey using this framework.

Further research is planned to fully tailor the concept of level analysis to the context of ISsec, and the framework will be applied to a comprehensive survey of ISsec literature. By drawing on this proposed framework, the data surrounding the research methodology of ISsec literature will be collected for the first time to shed light on the understudied area of the current ISsec research typology based on the paradigm, theory, method, and analysis. The results of this work will also be used to further refine the framework.

## 6   Conclusion

The growing interest in ISsec has prompted numerous research activities, but so far, these have been piecemeal and sporadic. Researchers have endeavoured to identify patterns or specific indications in the existing research by conducting literature reviews and surveys, but the lack of a systematic and coherent framework for examining previous research has so far hampered their efforts.

In light of this need, we propose a refined framework for examining ISsec research. The framework draws on previous studies for its four components: it adopts different typologies for research theory and method as the new criteria and incorporates research analysis from multilevel perspective, which was previously overlooked. We believe that this framework will provide effective support for future ISsec research, better guide the related research activities, and lay down the underpinnings of the exploration into the ISsec research typology.

# References

1. Hirschheim, R.: Information systems epistemology: an historical perspective. Res. Methods Inf. Syst. 13–35 (1985)
2. Brancheau, J.C., Janz, B.D., Wetherbe, J.C.: Key issues in information systems management: 1994–95 SIM Delphi results. MIS Q. 225–242 (1996)
3. BIS: 2013 information security breaches survey. Retrieved May 1, 2015, from https://www.gov.uk/government/uploads/system/uploads/attachment_data/file/191671/bis-13-p184es-2013-information-security-breaches-survey-executive-summary.pdf (2013)
4. Yeh, Q.-J., Chang, A.J.-T.: Threats and countermeasures for information system security: a cross-industry study. Inf. Manag. **44**(5), 480–491 (2007)
5. Siponen, M., Willison, R., Baskerville, R.: Power and practice in information systems security research. ICIS 2008 Proceedings: 26 (2008)
6. Baskerville, R.: Information systems security design methods: implications for information systems development. ACM Comput. Surv. (CSUR) **25**(4), 375–414 (1993)
7. Dhillon, G., Backhouse, J.: Current directions in IS security research: towards socio-organizational perspectives. Inf. Syst. J. **11**(2), 127–153 (2001)
8. Burrell, G., Morgan, G.: Sociological Paradigms and Organisational Analysis. Heinemann, London (1994)
9. Villarroel, R., Fernández-Medina, E., Piattini, M.: Secure information systems development—a survey and comparison. Comput. Secur. **24**(4), 308–321 (2005)
10. Siponen, M.: Analysis of modern IS security development approaches: towards the next generation of social and adaptable ISS methods. Inf. Organ. **15**(4), 339–375 (2005)
11. Laudan, L.: Science and Values. Cambridge University Press, Cambridge (1984)
12. Klein, K.J., Kozlowski, S.W.: Multilevel Theory, Research, and Methods in Organizations: Foundations, Extensions, and New Directions. Jossey-Bass, San Francisco (2000)
13. Hitt, M.A., Beamish, P.W., Jackson, S.E., Mathieu, J.E.: Building theoretical and empirical bridges across levels: multilevel research in management. Acad. Manag. J. **50**(6), 1385–1399 (2007)
14. Klein, K.J., Tosi, H., Cannella, A.A.: Multilevel theory building: benefits, barriers, and new developments. Acad. Manag. Rev. **24**(2), 248–253 (1999)
15. Klein, K.J., Dansereau, F., Hall, R.J.: Levels issues in theory development, data collection, and analysis. Acad. Manag. Rev. **19**(2), 195–229 (1994)
16. House, R., Rousseau, D.M., Thomashunt, M.: The meso paradigm—a framework for the integration of micro and macro organizational-behavior. Res. Organ. Behav. Annu. Series Anal. Essays Crit. Rev. **17**(1995), 71–114 (1995)
17. Rousseau, D.M.: Issues of level in organizational research: multi-level and cross-level perspectives. Res. Organ. Behav. **7**(1), 1–37 (1985)
18. Checkland, P.: Systems thinking, system practice. Wiley, New York (1981)
19. Iivari, J., Hirschheim, R., Klein, H.K.: A paradigmatic analysis contrasting information systems development approaches and methodologies. Inf. Syst. Res. **9**(2), 164–193 (1998)
20. Mingers, J.: Combining IS research methods: towards a pluralist methodology. Inf. Syst. Res. **12**(3), 240–259 (2001)

21. Orlikowski, W., J.Baroudi, J.J.: Studying information technology in organizations: research approaches and assumptions. Inf. Syst. Res. **2**(1): 1–28 (1991)
22. Chua, W.F.: Radical developments in accounting thought. Account. Rev. 601–632 (1986)
23. Gregor, S.: The nature of theory in information systems. MIS Q. 611–642 (2006)
24. Benbasat, I., Cash, J.I., Nunamaker, J.: The information systems research challenge, Harvard Business School, Boston (1989)
25. Alavi, M., Carlson, P., Brooke, G.: The ecology of MIS research: a twenty year status review. In: Proceedings of the Tenth International Conference on Information Systems, ACM (1989)
26. Klein, H.K., Myers, M.D.: A set of principles for conducting and evaluating interpretive field studies in information systems. MIS Q. 67–93 (1999)
27. von Alan, R.H., March, S.T., Park, J., Ram, S.: Design science in information systems research. MIS Q. **28**(1), 75–105 (2004)
28. Katz, D., Kahn, R.L.: The social psychology of organizations (1978)
29. Kozlowski, S.W., Klein, K.J.: A multilevel approach to theory and research in organizations: contextual, temporal, and emergent processes. In: Klein, K.J., Koslowski, S.W.J. (eds.) Multilevel Theory, Research, and Methods in Organizations (157–210). Jossey-Bass, San Francisco (2000)
30. Porter, L.W.: Forty years of organization studies: reflections from a micro perspective. Adm. Sci. Q. 262–269 (1996)
31. Thomson, M.E., von Solms, R.: Information security awareness: educating your users effectively. Inf. Manag. Comput. Secur. **6**(4), 167–173 (1998)
32. Siponen, M.T.: Five dimensions of information security awareness. Comput. Society **31**(2), 24–29 (2001)
33. Puhakainen, P.: A design theory for information security awareness. Faculty of Science, Department of Information Processing Science, University of Oulu. A 463 (2006)
34. D'Arcy, J., Hovav, A., Galletta, D.: User awareness of security countermeasures and its impact on information systems misuse: a deterrence approach. Inf. Syst. Res. **20**(1), 79–98 (2009)
35. Herath, T., Rao, H.R.: Encouraging information security behaviors in organizations: role of penalties, pressures and perceived effectiveness. Decis. Support Syst. **47**(2), 154–165 (2009)
36. Albrechtsen, E., Hovden, J.: Improving information security awareness and behaviour through dialogue, participation and collective reflection. An intervention study. Comput. Secur. **29**(4), 432–445 (2010)
37. Bulgurcu, B., Cavusoglu, H., Benbasat, I.: Information security policy compliance: an empirical study of rationality-based beliefs and information security awareness. MIS Q. **34**(3), 523–548 (2010)
38. Tariq, M.A., Brynielsson, J., Artman, H.: The security awareness paradox: a case study. In: 2014 IEEE/ACM International Conference on Advances in Social Networks Analysis and Mining (2014)
39. Gupta, A.K., Tesluk, P.E., Taylor, M.S.: Innovation at and across multiple levels of analysis. Organ. Sci. **18**(6), 885–897 (2007)

# An Agile Enterprise Architecture-Driven Model for Geographically Distributed Agile Development

Yehia Ibrahim Alzoubi and Asif Qumer Gill

**Abstract** Agile development is a highly collaborative environment, which requires active communication (i.e., effective and efficient communication) among stakeholders. Active communication in the geographically distributed agile development (GDAD) environment is difficult to achieve due to many challenges. Literature has reported that active communication plays a critical role in enhancing GDAD performance through reducing the cost and time of a project. However, little empirical evidence is known about how to study and establish active communication construct in GDAD in terms of its dimensions, determinants and effects on GDAD performance. To address this knowledge gap, this paper describes an enterprise architecture (EA) driven research model to identify and empirically examine the GDAD active communication construct. This model can be used by researchers and practitioners to examine the relationships among two dimensions of GDAD active communication (effectiveness and efficiency), one antecedent that can be controlled (agile EA), and four dimensions of GDAD performance (on-time completion, on-budget completion, software functionality and software quality).

**Keywords** Geographically distributed agile development · Communication effectiveness · Communication efficiency · Enterprise architecture

A prior version of this paper has been published in the ISD2015 Proceedings (http://aisel.aisnet.org/isd2014/proceedings2015/).

Y.I. Alzoubi (✉) · A.Q. Gill
School of Software, University of Technology Sydney, Sydney, Australia
e-mail: yehia.i.alzoubi@student.uts.edu.au

A.Q. Gill
e-mail: asif.gill@uts.edu.au

© Springer International Publishing Switzerland 2016
D. Vogel et al. (eds.), *Transforming Healthcare Through Information Systems*,
Lecture Notes in Information Systems and Organisation 17,
DOI 10.1007/978-3-319-30133-4_5

# 1   Introduction

Agile methods have been introduced to address a number of issues related to project development and delivery, such as over-budget or behind schedule projects, and not meeting customer's needs and expectations [1]. Agile methods emerged over a period of time to increasingly influence future trends in software development in both the local and distributed contexts [2]. GDAD refers to the agile development that includes teams or/and team members distributed over different locations and time zones [3]. GDAD faces many challenges. The most noticeable challenge is the communication and knowledge sharing between dispersed teams and customers [4–6].

Communication is defined as the process of exchanging information between senders and receivers [7]. Communication can also be defined as a way to manage relationships between developers and consumers [8]. These definitions draw our attention to the importance and effectiveness of communication between the parties included in agile development. However, agile methods promise faster develop-ment thus improving the communication efficiency too [9]. Thus, agile methods require effective and efficient communication (i.e., active communication) among stakeholders to achieve the highest software quality and customer satisfaction [2, 10]. Herbsleb and Mockus [11] divide communication in agile software development into two general types; formal and informal communication. Formal communication can be defined as the explicit clear communication such as the agile requirements backlog and card walls [11]. Informal communication refers to per-sonal peer-oriented conversation among developers which takes place outside the official structure and sometimes without the knowledge of management [11]. Informal communication helps in filling and correcting mistakes quickly, which supports and ensures agile principles [11].

To overcome the uncertainty and changeable customer's requirements, active communication is considered vital in a co-located agile development team. The importance of active communication is greater in GDAD due to less chances of informal face-to-face communication [2]. In GDAD, active communication is harder to achieve due to many challenges such as differences in language, culture, distance, time-zone, architecture used, management process, and communication infrastructure between distributed teams [12].

It has been reported in the literature that active communication may enhance GDAD design and quality by reducing the project development time and cost [9]. The empirical knowledge on the subject seems to be scarce. To address this knowledge gap, there is a need to empirically examine how active communication can be achieved to enhance GDAD performance [5]. This paper addresses this important gap and proposes an agile EA driven model for enabling GDAD active communication and examining how this model can enhance GDAD performance. The aim of this paper is to uncover the relationships between the agile EA, GDAD communication and GDAD performance. This paper is an incremental output of our ongoing research in the area of agile enterprise architecture and GDAD communication.

The paper is structured as follows: Sect. 2 discusses the research method. Section 3 presents the theoretical foundation. Section 4 discusses the agile EA driven GDAD communication research model and hypotheses. Section 5 discusses the preliminary evaluation of research model. Section 6 discusses the research findings, limitations and future directions before concluding.

## 2 Research Method

This section describes the overall research methodology that we are applying to iteratively develop and evaluate the proposed model. We are applying an integrated multi-method approach that uses both qualitative and quantitative techniques [13]. This approach consists of three phases: (1) building the research model, which includes two stages: build the theoretical research model (i.e., agile EA driven GDAD communication model) from the literature review and preliminary model evaluation, (2) survey data collection, which includes two stages: conducting pilot study (i.e. measurement validation) and analyzing the main survey data (i.e., hypothesis testing), and (3) final model evaluation by conducting semi-structured interviews using a case study approach. Using this multi-method approach helps in addressing limitations for both qualitative and quantitative methods by providing the objectivity of the statistics and deeper understanding of the study context [13]. The scope of this paper is limited to phases 1 of this large multi-year project. In the first stage of phase 1, the agile EA driven GDAD communication model was built based on the previous related literature. In the second stage of phase 1, preliminary model evaluation was conducted by involving five experts from both academia and industry. This paper presents the refined version of the model for further feedback from the research community. This preliminary evaluation is done to identify any issues and get directions before proceeding further in the research.

## 3 Theoretical Foundations

This section discusses the relevant literature and identifies three constructs of the proposed agile EA driven GDAD communication model: agile EA (including one antecedent or independent variable: agile EA), GDAD active communication (including two dimensions or dependent variables: efficiency and effectiveness), and GDAD performance (including four dimensions or dependent variables: on-time completion, on-budget completion, software functionality and software quality). Table 1 synthesizes the literature review and presents the resultant agile EA driven GDAD communication model variables.

This research adopts a challenge driven approach. Firstly, we had conducted a detailed systematic literature review to identify the GDAD communication challenges [5]. Seven challenges categories were identified in the systematic literature review: (1) *People Differences* (refer to four communication challenges: cultural

**Table 1** The agile EA driven GDAD communication model variables

| Variable | Literature | Relevant Definitions/Concepts/Ideas |
|---|---|---|
| Agile enterprise architecture | [14] | • Agile EA should be a team effort following the strategy of "everyone owns the architecture" where big up-front design is not required and a minimum documentation is required |
| | [15] | • Agile EA describes the overall structural, behavioral, social, technological, and facility elements of an enterprise |
| | [16] | • The architecture is an important communication tool<br>• The architecture is a coordination mechanism in multi-site development |
| | [17] | • Architecture can be assumed as a language metaphor, where architecture description about structures and solutions serve as communication enabler between different stakeholders |
| | [18] | • Using architecture was perceived as delivering large volumes of rich information in global sites and enhances active communication through a common vocabulary |
| Communication efficiency | [19] | • Efficiency concerns with short manufacturing times, lead times, cycle times and work times |
| | [11] | • Splitting work across sites slows the work down<br>• Enhance communication efficiency through timely communication and right people to communicate with |
| | [20] | • Efficiency relates to the time, cost, resources, or effort associated with software team responses |
| | [21] | • Efficiency refers to doing things right of any task, even if it is not important to the job, that meets all the standards of time, quality, etc. |
| | [22] | • Rapid communication is a success factor of GDAD practices<br>• Larger team might pose great hindrance to fast communication |
| Communication effectiveness | [23] | • GDAD requires effective communication (e.g., teleconference) and instant feedback from the customer |
| | [24] | • Communication effectiveness means minimal disruption, waiting time, and misunderstanding to get the information<br>• Communication effectiveness requires immediate feedback which reduces waiting time, helps team members to address problems, and minimize clashes |
| | [25] | • Communication effectiveness facilitates knowledge transfer rapidly between team members, allows team members to understand the requirements from clients, and helps team members perform development activities efficiently<br>• Communication effectiveness can be increased by reducing the effect of communication challenges such as time-zone differences and language barrier, and increasing effective formal and informal communication |

(continued)

**Table 1** (continued)

| Variable | Literature | Relevant Definitions/Concepts/Ideas |
|---|---|---|
| | [11] | • Communication effectiveness refers to delivering a complete, adequate and accurate message<br>• Communication effectiveness requires communication frequency and coordination between GDAD team |
| | [21] | • Effectiveness accounts for doing the right things. Refers just to the tasks that are important to the job, even if they are completed without meeting standards of time, quality, etc. |
| On-time completion | [26] | • Delivering software project on time |
| | [20] | • The extent to which a software project meets its baseline goals for duration |
| | [21] | • Accounts for meeting datelines, overtime needed to complete the work, and other time related issues |
| On-budget completion | [26] | • Delivering software project within estimated cost and effort |
| | [20] | • The extent to which a software project meets its baseline goals for cost |
| | [27] | • The extent to which a software project is completed within or near the estimated budget |
| Software functionality | [26] | • Meeting all requirements and objectives |
| | [20] | • The extent to which the delivered software system meets its functional goals, user needs, and technical requirements |
| | [27] | • The extent to which a software project meets its technical goals |
| Software quality | [26] | • Delivering good product or project outcome |
| | [26] | • Achieving high standards in terms of the software and supporting documentation produced, and the development team |
| | [27] | • The extent to which the project performance is improved |
| | [22] | • Productivity, customer satisfaction, business processes, and functionality can be perceived as quality criteria |

difference, people attitude, language, and trust), (2) *Distance Differences* (refer to two communication challenges: different time zones and different geographical areas), (3) *Team Issues* (refer to four challenges: team size, team distribution, cross-team work, and cross-team communication), (4) *Technology Issues* (refer to four challenges: communication tools, infrastructures, communication bandwidth, and communication cost), (5) *Architectural Issues* (refer to four challenges: architectures used, organizational structure, managerial structure, and project domain), (6) *Process Issues* (refer to three challenges: process, control, and commitment-level to communication), and (7) *Customer Communication* (refers to involvement and transparency with customer). We focused our research on agile EA (see (5) *Architectural Issues*), which is the least investigated area in the context of GDAD. This research adopts an agile EA driven approach as a potential facilitator and enhancer of communication in GDAD environment. Agile EA seems more appropriate and fit to the people driven and light-weight agile ways of working [28], and therefore, it has been adopted for this research.

## 3.1 GDAD Active Communication: Efficiency and Effectiveness

Communication between developers and with customers is core to the agile development [10]. Agile software development approaches have been introduced as the alternative methods to the traditional "heavyweight" methods that do not have the enough ability to address the current issues such as development time and cost, and respond to uncertain changeable customer's requirements [3, 29, 30]. To overcome these issues, agile development focuses on the role of people and communication. It values people and interactions over processes and tools, and customer collaboration over contract negotiation [10]. It promotes close collaboration and communication between empowered development teams and customers [10].

As shown in Table 1, prior literature provides various theoretical concepts of communication efficiency and effectiveness. There is a common theme underlying the various definitions and descriptions in that communication is generally defined in terms of exchanging the adequate information in short time [21–25].

Furthermore, it appears that prior literature tends to view communication as consisting of two important elements that correspond to our conceptualization of the two communication dimensions: communication efficiency and communication effectiveness. Efficiency deals with short manufacturing times, lead times, cycle times and work times [19]. Efficiency relates to time, cost, resources, or effort associated with communication [20]. It also refers to doing things (i.e. any task) correctly, even if it is not important to the job (i.e. the task is completed meeting all the standards of time, quality, etc.) [21]. Effectiveness concerns with the practices or ways to effectively respond to market and customer demands [19]. Communication effectiveness means as little as possible disruption, minimal waiting time to get the required information and minimal chances of misunderstanding [24]. It also refers to doing the right things just to the tasks which are important to the job, even if they are completed without meeting standards of time, quality, etc. [21]. To avoid any confusion in the definitions of effectiveness and efficiency from the previous literature, we define communication efficiency as delivering a message to a receiver with high quality and with minimal time, cost, effort, and resources required to establish communication. Moreover, we define communication effectiveness as delivering a message to the receiver who understands it as it was intended with minimal disruption and misunderstanding, even if it takes a long time.

## 3.2 Agile Enterprise Architecture

The EA is defined as "a blueprint that describes the overall structural, behavioral, social, technological, and facility elements of an enterprise's operating environment that share common goals and principles" [15, p. 1]. Agile enterprise is defined as "an entity is said to be an agile enterprise when an enterprise is responsive (scans, senses and reacts appropriately to expected and unexpected changes), flexible (adapts to expected or unexpected change at any time), speedy (accommodates expected or unexpected changes rapidly), lean (focuses on reducing waste and cost without compromising on quality), and learning (focuses on enterprise fitness, improvement and innovation)" [15, p. 3]. Hence, agile EA can be defined as a blueprint that describes the overall structural, behavioral, social, technological, and facility elements of an enterprise's operating environment that share common goals and principles with the ability of responsiveness, flexibility, speediness, leanness, and learning [15, 19, 28]. Unlike traditional process-focused heavy architecture frameworks (e.g., Zachman [31]), agile architecture frameworks (e.g., The Gill Framework® [32]) provide human-centric, align to agile principles, and adaptive capabilities to adapting, defining, operating, managing and supporting an agile EA.

Agile principles make it clear that the best architectures, requirements, and designs emerge from self-organizing teams [10]. Moreover, business people and agile developers must work together daily throughout the project [10]. These two principles work well for a small co-located agile team where developers work side by side and communicate face-to-face with business people [33]. This helps developers and business people to work out the best project architecture and design through effective collaboration [33]. However, in GDAD environment, the opportunity for this effective collaborative and continuous communication among developers and with business people is limited due to many barriers, as discussed above [12]. This situation becomes even more challenging when the organization deploys many GDAD teams that need to work simultaneously on different dependent features or projects. In such complex GDAD environment, efficient and effective communication between different silo GDAD teams is required for alignment and continuous delivery of working features or projects.

GDAD teams need to be continuously communicating with each other due to changing of their and other dependent project(s) architectures and requirements for alignment [33]. This could be achieved with some sort of overall holistic and integrated EA [34]. Using holistic and integrated agile EA along with available communication tools may facilitate and enhance communication between GDAD teams. However, unlike traditional process-focused EA approaches, which are often considered too heavy for agile development, agile development requires an adaptive people-focused EA to provide the integrated shared view of the enterprise projects for GDAD teams [14]. This paper proposes one such agile EA driven GDAD communication n model. The holistic agile EA may serve as a common information model and integrated shared view for enabling clear communication among GDAD teams [16, 28]. The agile EA driven GDAD communication approach can enable communication via different architectural views at different enterprise project management levels [4, 32]: (1) distributed teams share the "project solution architecture view", (2) different projects share the "program solution architecture view", (3) the same is applied to the holistic "enterprise solution architecture view", which can have "N" number of program architectures, (4) each architecture updates the architecture above, and (5) all architectures are then updated and shared from the holistic agile EA integrated shared view. This ensures that all distributed stakeholders are updated with the latest changes (i.e. project or program changes, dependencies within and across distributed projects) [34].

## 3.3   GDAD Performance

Researchers have diverse interpretations of software development performance. Some have referred to it as a project success [22, 27]. A project is assumed to be successful if it is completed within or close to the success criteria boundary such as the estimated time/schedule, budget/cost, scope (functionality) and acceptable level of quality [22]. Time, budget and quality are the key components of any project's success [22]. Others have referred to it as project effectiveness [35, 36]. Project is assumed to be effective if it meets the speed, schedule and efficiency [36]. Aspects related to effectiveness are project duration, effort and quality [35].

Both traditional software development literature and agile literature have looked at software development performance dimensions as on-time completion, on-budget completion, and software functionality [20, 37]. This study adopts these three dimensions of the software development performance; however, we argue that quality is an important dimension of performance. Therefore, this study refers to on-time completion, on-budget completion, functionality and quality as the four performance dimensions [26] (see Table 1), which can be depicted in Fig. 1. On-time completion refers to the extent to which a software project meets its baseline goals for duration [20]. On-budget completion refers to the extent to which a software project meets its

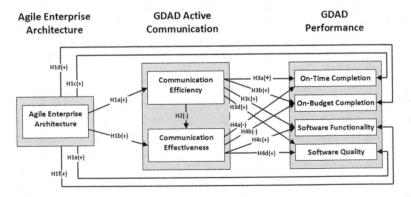

**Fig. 1** The agile EA driven GDAD communication model

baseline goals for cost [20]. Functionality refers to the extent to which the delivered software project meets its functional scope goals, user needs, and technical requirements [20]. Quality refers to delivering a good working product [26].

# 4 The Agile EA Driven GDAD Communication Model

The refined and updated agile EA driven GDAD communication model and related hypotheses (based on theoretical review and the preliminary expert evaluation) are shown in Fig. 1. The central construct of the research model is GDAD active communication. The relationships and hypotheses between the constructs of the model are discussed in the following sections.

## 4.1 Effect of Agile EA on GDAD Active Communication

Agile EA as an integrated shared view may provide a comprehensive view (i.e. holistic understanding and knowledge) and a common language for GDAD teams' members [16, 38]. This may enhance GDAD active communication and overcome problems related to different spoken languages and different cultures [39]. As a result, communication efficiency and effectiveness may be increased. Using EA in distributed development was found to provide rich information source in large volumes [18]. This indicates that agile EA can be used as a communication mechanism enabler [18], and as a communication tool between different GDAD stakeholders [16]. Moreover, by using agile EA, as an integrated shared view (as proposed in this paper), GDAD developers can coordinate their work through interfaces of their components such that each component can be developed separately. This means that the frequency of communication as well as considering the developments of other components are decreased [16]. However, agile EA artifact should be communicated (e.g., by architect), both informally and through formal descriptions, to all GDAD stakeholders [16]. Without adequate communication and common understanding about EA among GDAD stakeholders, a project may fail technically and organizationally [17]. In a nutshell, we propose that agile EA may enhance GDAD active communication. Therefore, we propose:

**Hypothesis 1a** Agile Enterprise Architecture positively affects the efficiency of the GDAD communication.
**Hypothesis 1b** Agile Enterprise Architecture positively affects effectiveness of the GDAD communication.

## 4.2 Effect of Agile EA on GDAD Performance

Agile EA is important for GDAD project [14]. It draws from a uniform infrastructure, platform, application, and communicates the architecture value and status with all stakeholders [40]. Moreover, it improves implementation consistency and reduces the number of errors by providing the basis for architecture rules to involved teams [38]. Agile EA may enhance software performance as it is the placeholder for software quality, modifiability, security, and reliability [38, 40]. This means that EA may have a positive impact on the GDAD performance, which means increasing the agility of GDAD project, according to agile principles [10]. Therefore, we propose:

**Hypothesis 1c** Agile Enterprise Architecture positively influences on-time completion of GDAD project.
**Hypothesis 1d** Agile Enterprise Architecture positively influences on-budget completion of GDAD project.
**Hypothesis 1e** Agile Enterprise Architecture positively influences GDAD project quality.
**Hypothesis 1f** Agile Enterprise Architecture positively influences GDAD project functionality.

## 4.3 Relationship Between GDAD Communication Efficiency and Effectiveness

Considering the impacts of time, cost and effort on communication, GDAD team tends to first choose what and how much they would communicate. This choice in turn affects communication effectiveness. Furthermore, the extensively engaged GDAD team leads to more effectiveness of the communication [25]. Moreover, due to GDAD communication challenges, the message may not be received as it was effectively intended. The shortness may be insufficient to deliver clear message. In other words, efficiency may decrease the effectiveness of GDAD communication. Therefore, we propose

**Hypothesis 2** GDAD communication efficiency negatively affects effectiveness of the GDAD communication.

## 4.4 Effect of GDAD Active Communication on GDAD Performance

The whole idea behind agility is being fast (e.g., fast delivery, fast communication). Fast communication and informal communication may lead to fast responding to customer requirements, which results in high agile development performance [22, 30, 41]. Delays in identifying project impacts, dependencies, and resultant changes in GDAD environment may lead to longer development duration and extra cost. If the efficiency of GDAD communication is high, the amount of extra time and costs required for handling ongoing changes is minimal. This may reduce the additional time and cost, and meet the assigned time and budget targets [20]. Furthermore, as the GDAD team repeatedly implements responses to similar types of requirement changes, communication efficiency as well as optimizing and perfection of their work increase. Therefore, efficient GDAD communication is expected to effectively satisfy user requirements, which may result in high software functionality. Moreover, efficient GDAD communication may result in faster response to project changes [30]. This may help in delivering better working system (i.e. better system quality). Therefore, we propose

**Hypothesis 3a** Communication efficiency positively influences on-time completion of GDAD project.
**Hypothesis 3b** Communication efficiency positively influences on-budget completion of GDAD project.
**Hypothesis 3c** Communication efficiency positively influences GDAD project functionality.
**Hypothesis 3d** Communication efficiency positively influences GDAD project quality.

Effective communication plays a vital role in understanding customer's requirements and feedback. Yet, the higher communication effectiveness comes at the price of considerably longer time and higher cost, while the shorter and faster communication come at a price of a noticeably lower effectiveness [35]. We posit that effective communication causes time and cost overruns. To effectively communicate about many different customer requirements and requirements' changes, GDAD team may need new resources and capabilities or reconfigure existing resources and capabilities [20]. This requires a considerable amount of extra time and cost [20]. Furthermore, we posit that effective communication increases system functionality and quality. That is, communication about customer's requirements and requirements' changes helps in the correctness of system configuration; improve design and product quality [23]. The functionality and quality of the system will not satisfy "up-to-date" customer needs if the team fails to embrace important changes [20]. Therefore, we propose

**Hypothesis 4a** Communication effectiveness negatively influences on-time completion of GDAD project.
**Hypothesis 4b** Communication effectiveness negatively influences on-budget completion of GDAD project.
**Hypothesis 4c** Communication effectiveness positively influences GDAD project functionality.
**Hypothesis 4d** Communication effectiveness positively influences GDAD project quality.

## 5 Preliminary Evaluation of Research Model

Following the recommendation by Gable [13], the initial evaluation of the proposed model was conducted by involving five experts from both academia and industry. Preliminary field interviews were conducted with 5 experts in agile development.

Three of them were from agile development industry; a Scrum Master, a developer and an architect. Two of them worked as agile developers and now are assistant professors teaching agile development and agile enterprise architecture subjects. Two experts were asked the questions during 60-min semi-structured face-to-face interviews, and three experts were emailed the model and questions [13]. The asked questions included:

- Is the design of the model clear, well thought out and easy to understand?
- Does it provide the necessary (relevant and important) constructs?
- Does it provide the necessary (relevant and important) relationships between the constructs?
- Does it provide the necessary (relevant and important) hypothesis?
- Is it suitable for its intended purpose?

The feedback supports the model design and its understandability, its constructs and relationships between different variables, and its suitability for the purpose of research. One expert wrote: *"I think the model has been rigorously built and the relationships between different variables have been clearly identified"*. The feedback supports the role of agile EA and the role of the two communication dimensions; efficiency and effectiveness in GDAD. One expert mentioned: *"Investigating agile EA role in the distributed agile environment seems to be very interesting and has a lot of potential"*. Another expert mentioned: *"when we talk about communication, we are assuming quick and focused message"*. We estimated some disagreement on the definitions of functionality and quality variables from the interviews. Some experts refer to functionality as a part of quality. One expert mentioned: *"...functionality is a part of quality since without achieving its functionality, software cannot be assumed of high quality"*. However, it is envisioned that functionality and quality are different concepts at this stage (subject to further research) so we included them in the model as separate variables. Moreover, a direct relationship between agile EA and GDAD performance was included in the model since some feedback assume that there is direct effect of agile EA on project performance. One expert suggested that: *"I believe EA have more effect on project performance than on communication"*. Considering all feedback, the updated model was sent via email to the same above expert group for evaluation. Based on the second feedback, we validated the Agile EA driven GDAD communication model (Fig. 1) for further research.

## 6   Discussion, Limitations and Future Directions

This paper introduced the agile EA driven GDAD communication model. This model includes three constructs: agile EA, GDAD active communication, and GDAD performance. These constructs and their variables are presented in this paper based on the literature review and the expert evaluation. The central construct is GDAD active communication, which includes two dependent variables:

efficiency and effectiveness. While efficiency refers to fast communication, effectiveness refers to quality of communication. Agile EA includes one independent variable: agile EA. GDAD performance includes four dependent variables: on-time completion, on-budget completion, software functionality and software quality. Software functionality and quality are two different concepts, as discussed in this paper. While functionality refers to meeting the goals and requirements of software project, quality refers to good working software.

This model provides a new perspective of agile EA as an integrated shared view to support GDAD communication, which is currently deemed as a gap in literature. Scaling agile approaches for GDAD environment requires scaling GDAD communication at the enterprise level to supporting multiple GDAD teams, projects and their alignment. Agile EA as an integrated shared view may provide a common language for GDAD teams' members. This means that agile EA may facilitate and enhance communication in GDAD environment. Since communication is the core of agile development, enhancing GDAD communication results in enhancing GDAD agility and performance [9]. The findings of this paper are expected to have significant implications on GDAD practitioners and academics through using agile EA as a GDAD communication enabler or tool.

Similar to any other study, this study has some limitations. One may argue that this study investigates only the effect of agile EA on GDAD and does not investigate the other communication challenges categories. This study is specially focused on the potential perspective of using agile EA, which has not been discussed before and marks the need for theoretical and empirical research. Moreover, some of the categories of communication challenges (i.e., People Differences, Distance Differences, and Technology Issues) have been paid too much attention in the previous literature. Also, studying Customer Communication is out of the range of the paper, as our research focus is only on enhancing communication inter and intra geographically distributed teams working on different dependent projects in GDAD environment. In addition, we assume that Team Issues and Process Issues challenges categories will be enhanced as a result of using agile EA in GDAD. However, the above limitation keeps the door open to investigate other challenges categories such as Team Issues and Process Issues. In a nutshell, more empirical research is needed in this field.

# 7 Conclusions

This paper presented an agile EA driven GDAD communication model based on the literature review and preliminary evaluation. This paper draws our attention to the importance of studying agile EA and its effect on GDAD communication and performance. The proposed updated model includes three important constructs and relationships: agile EA, GDAD active communication, and GDAD performance. These constructs were rigorously identified from the previous literature and verified through preliminary evaluation. This study is one of the initial efforts to examine agile EA effect on GDAD communication and GDAD performance. We believe that many questions are yet to be answered in this area. We hope this study will serve as a starting point for developing and testing theories for guiding communication in GDAD environment so that organizations can effectively build and sustain communication that will ultimately improve their GDAD performance.

# References

1. Balijepally, V., Mahapatra, R., Nerur, S., Price, K.H.: Are two heads better than one for software development? The productivity paradox of pair programming. MISQ, pp. 91–118 (2009)
2. Gill, A.Q.: Distributed agile development: applying a coverage analysis approach to the evaluation of a communication technology assessment tool. Int. J. e-Collab (IJeC) **11**, 57–76 (2015)
3. Highsmith, J.A.I.: Adaptive software development: a collaborative approach to managing complex systems. Dorset House Publishing, New York (2000)
4. Agerfalk, P., Fitzgerald, B., Slaughter, S.: Flexible and distributed information systems development: state of the art and research challenges. Inf. Syst. Res. **20**, 317–328 (2009)
5. Korkala, M., Pikkarainen, M., Conboy, K.: Distributed agile development: a case study of customer communication challenges. In: Abrahamsson, P., Marchesi, M., Maurer, F. (eds.) XP 2009, LNBIP, vol. 31, pp. 161–167. Springer, Heidelberg (2009)
6. Vidgen, R., Wang, X.: Coevolving systems and the organization of agile software development. Inf. Syst. Res. **20**, 355–376 (2009)
7. McQuail, D.: Mass communication theory: an introduction. Sage Publications, Thousand Oaks (1987)
8. Malone, T.W., Crowston, K.: The interdisciplinary study of coordination. ACM Comput. Surv. **26**, 87–119 (1994)
9. Pikkarainen, M., Haikara, J., Salo, O., Abrahamsson, P., Still, J.: The impact of agile practices on communication in software development. Empir. Softw. Eng. **13**, 303–337 (2008)
10. Agile Manifesto: Manifesto for agile software development. http://www.agilemanifesto.org
11. Herbsleb, J.D., Mockus, A.: An empirical study of speed and communication in globally distributed software development. IEEE Trans. Softw. Eng. **29**, 481–494 (2003)
12. Alzoubi, Y.I., Gill, A.Q.: Agile global software development communication challenges: a systematic review. In: 18th Pacific Asia Conference on Information Systems, China (2014)
13. Gable, G.G.: Integrating case study and survey research methods: an example in information systems. Eur. J. Inf. Syst. **3**, 112–126 (1994)
14. Ambler, S.: Agile Enterprise Architecture. http://www.agiledata.org
15. Gill, A.Q.: Towards the development of an adaptive enterprise service system model. In: 19th Americas Conference on Information Systems, pp. 1–9. Chicago, Illinois (2013)
16. Ovaska, P., Rossi, M., Marttiin, P.: Architecture as a coordination tool in multi-site software development. Softw. Process. Improv. Pract. **8**, 233–247 (2003)
17. Smolander, K.: Four metaphors of architecture in software organizations: finding out the meaning of architecture in practice. In: International Symposium on Empirical Software Engineering, pp. 211–221. IEEE (2002)
18. Svensson, R.B., Aurum, A., Paech, B., Gorschek, T., Sharma, D.: Software architecture as a means of communication in a globally distributed software development context. In: Dieste, O., Jedlitschka, A., Juristo, N. (eds.) PROFES 2012, LNCS, vol. 7343, pp. 175–189. Springer, Heidelberg (2012)
19. Franke, U., Ekstedt, M., Lagerström, R., Saat, J., Winter, R.: Trends in enterprise architecture practice—a survey. In: Proper, E. et al. (eds.) TEAR 2010, LNBIP, vol. 70, pp. 16–29. Springer, Heidelberg (2010)

20. Lee, G., Xia, W.: Toward agile: an integrated analysis of quantitative and qualitative field data. MISQ **34**, 87–114 (2010)
21. Melo, C., Cruzes, D.S., Kon, F., Conradi, R.: Agile team perceptions of productivity factors. In: Agile Conference, pp. 57–66. IEEE (2011)
22. Misra, S.C., Kumar, V., Kumar, U.: Identifying some important success factors in adopting agile software development practices. J. Syst. Softw. **82**, 1869–1890 (2009)
23. Bhalerao, S., Ingle, M.: Analyzing the modes of communication in agile practices. In: 3rd IEEE International Conference on Computer Science and Information Technology, pp. 391–395. IEEE Press, New York (2010)
24. Cannizzo, F., Marcionetti, G., Moser, P.: Evolution of the tools and practices of a large distributed agile team. In: Agile Conference 08, pp. 513–518. IEEE (2008)
25. Dorairaj, S., Noble, J., Malik, P.: Effective communication in distributed agile software development teams. In: Sillitti, A., et al. (Eds.) XP 2011, LNBIP, vol. 77, pp. 102–116. Springer, Heidelberg (2011)
26. Chow, T., Cao, D.-B.: A survey study of critical success factors in agile software projects. J. Syst. Softw. **81**, 961–971 (2008)
27. Mahaney, R.C., Lederer, A.L.: The effect of intrinsic and extrinsic rewards for developers on information systems project success. Proj. Manag. J. **37**, 42–54 (2006)
28. Gill, A.Q.: Adaptive cloud enterprise architecture. World Scientific (2015b)
29. Beck, K.: Extreme programming explained. Addison-Wesley, Boston (2000)
30. Cockburn, A.: Agile software development: the cooperative game. Addison-Wesley, Harlow (2007)
31. Zachman, J.A.: A framework for information systems architecture. IBM Syst. J. **26**, 276–292 (1987)
32. Gill, A.Q.: The Gill Framework®. http://www.aqgill.com/adoms
33. Fruhling, A., Vreede, G.-J.D.: Field experiences with eXtreme programming: developing an emergency response system. J. Manag. Info. Syst. **22**, 39–68 (2006)
34. Alzoubi, Y.I., Gill, A.Q., Al-Ani, A.: Distributed agile development communication: an agile architecture driven framework. J. Softw. **10**, 681–694 (2015)
35. Dyba, T., Arisholm, E., Sjoberg, D.I., Hannay, J.E., Shull, F.: Are two heads better than one? On the effectiveness of pair programming. IEEE Softw. **24**, 12–15 (2007)
36. Jiang, J., Klein, G.: Software development risks to project effectiveness. J. Syst. Softw. **52**, 3–10 (2000)
37. Aladwani, A.M.: An integrated performance model information systems projects. J. Manag. Inf. Syst. **19**, 185–210 (2002)
38. Bass, L., Kazman, R.: Architecture-based development. Technical Report (No. CMU/SEI-99-TR-007, ESC-TR-99-007), Carnegie Mellon Software Engineering Institute (1999)
39. Ambler, S.: Choose the Best Communication Technique. http://disciplinedagiledelivery.com
40. Madison, J.: Agile architecture interactions. IEEE Softw. **27**, 41–48 (2010)
41. Boehm, B., Turner, R.: Balancing agility and discipline: a guide for the perplexed. Addison-Wesley Professional (2003)

# Community-Based Message Opportunistic Transmission

Sheng Zhang, Pengliu Tan, Xiaoling Bao, William Wei Song
and Xiaodong Liu

**Abstract** A Mobile Social Networks (MSN) is a kind of opportunistic network, which is composed of numerous mobile nodes with social characteristic. By now, the prevalent community-based routing algorithms mainly choose the optimal social characteristic node to forward messages, however they rarely consider the effects of community distribution on mobile nodes and time-varying characteristics of network. These algorithms usually lead to a high consumption of network resources and a low successful delivery ratio if they are used directly in mobile social networks. In order to solve this problem, we build a time-varying community-based network model, and propose a community-aware message opportunistic transmission algorithm (CMOT) in this paper. For inter-community messages transmission, the CMOT chooses an optimal community path by comparing the community transmission probability. In local communities, messages are forwarded according to the encounter probability between nodes. The simulation results show that, in comparison with classical routing algorithms, such as PRoPHET, MaxProp, Spray and Wait, and CMTS, the CMOT can improve the successful delivery ratio of messages and reduce network overhead obviously.

A prior version of this paper has been published in the ISD2015 Proceedings (http://aisel.aisnet.org/isd2014/proceedings2015/).

S. Zhang (✉) · X. Bao · X. Liu
School of Information Engineering, Nanchang Hangkong University, Nanchang, China
e-mail: zwxzs168@126.com

X. Bao
e-mail: bxl007315@sina.com

X. Liu
e-mail: technology12@163.com

P. Tan
Internet of Things Institute, Nanchang Hangkong University, Nanchang, China
e-mail: pltan@nchu.edu.cn

W.W. Song
Business Intelligence and Informatics, Dalarna University, Borlänge, Sweden
e-mail: wso@du.se

© Springer International Publishing Switzerland 2016
D. Vogel et al. (eds.), *Transforming Healthcare Through Information Systems*,
Lecture Notes in Information Systems and Organisation 17,
DOI 10.1007/978-3-319-30133-4_6

79

**Keywords** Mobile social networks · Message opportunistic transmission · Transmission probability · Encounter probability

# 1 Introduction

A Mobile Social Network (MSN) is a special type of Opportunistic Networks (ON), built on the concepts of Delay-Tolerant Networks (DTN) and Mobile Ad hoc Networks (MANET) [1]. Due to the increasing use of short-distance wireless mobile devices (such as smart phones, smart bracelets, Apple Watches, iPads, etc.), the direct communication and data sharing for each other are becoming more and more convenient [2]. The typical applications of mobile social networks are booming, such as pocket switched networks (PSN) [3], mobile vehicular networks (VN) [4], and wireless sensor networks [5].

In MSNs, the communication between nodes shows intermittent connectivity due to the nodes' moving. Therefore, it is not possible to run the traditional routing protocols; the MSN only depends on the encounter opportunity among nodes to forward messages. Consequently, the "Storage-Carry-Forward" strategy is usually used to deliver messages in MSNs. In addition, the nodes generally tend to congregate together according to social relations in MSNs, this shows community feathers. All nodes form various natural communities which have respective regions divided by the real or logical boundaries. The nodes are much active in itself community, while they hardly move to other communities. There are just a few nodes which can visit other communities according to their interest, they are likely to set up ties between different communities. In this case, efficiently forwarding messages from source node to destination node is challenging.

# 2 Related Work

Message forwarding in MSNs has been research extensively. Some typical message forwarding algorithms, such as Epidemic based on multi-copy replication [6], Spray and Wait [7], Spray and Focus [8], PRoPHET [9], MaxProp [10], and CMTS [11], have been developed. These inject a large amount of message copies into the network to improve the successful delivery ratio and reduce transmission delay. However, too many copies will consume a lot of network resources. In addition, these algorithms do not consider social characteristics.

At present, some message transmission algorithms with social characteristics have been proposed. Hui and Crowcroft [12] put forward a routing label strategy that takes advantage of the social structure to transmit messages. It creates a label for each node telling others about its affiliation. In the same community, the node with high encounter probability will get a high opportunity to deliver successful the messages. But this routing performance is significantly degraded when the nodes do not mix well or messages have a short TTL (time-to-live). Relatedly, Hui et al. [13] proposed Bubble Rap, a social-based message forwarding algorithm in a DTN. In this algorithm, each node is designed to have global or local ranking. The messages are forwarded to nodes that have high global ranking until a node in the destination's community is found. Subsequently, the messages are forwarded to nodes that have higher local ranking within the destination's community. But the drawback of this algorithm is a low message successful delivery ratio and a high network delay in single-copy message transmission.

Xiao et al. [14] proposed a single-copy routing algorithm CAOR based on community-awareness. In this algorithm, mobile nodes with a common interest autonomously form a community, the frequently visited location is called their common home. The nodes with high centrality act as the home of their community. The whole network is composed of some overlapped star-topology communities. The CAOR converts the routing between nodes into the routing between community homes at first. Then, using a reverse Dijkstra algorithm, the CAOR obtains an optimal relay set for each home to determine the optimal relays. Each home only forwards the message to the nodes which belong to its optimal relay set, and ignores other relays. However, the time complexity of CAOR is associated with the number of community. When the network scale becomes large and the number of community increases, the CAOR decreases the successful delivery ratio and increases network overhead.

In addition, Zhu [15] proposed a location-based routing to measure nodes' social relations by location similarity. When the nodes access similar locations, they own a close social relations and have high encounter probability. The messages are only forwarded among the close nodes. Bulut and Szymanski [16] proposed friendship-based routing in Delay Tolerant Mobile Social Networks. A group of nodes that have a directly or indirectly close relationship form a time-varying friendship community, and a message is only forwarded to the node that belongs to the same community.

All above messages forwarding strategies usually select the nodes with the optimal sociality to deliver, but they do not consider the fact that the distribution of communities exert influence on nodes mobility.

In this paper, we build a time-varying community-based network model and propose a community-aware message opportunistic transmission algorithm (CMOT). We assume that there are $m$ communities for $n$ nodes in MSN. The $m$ communities are empty at first. After the network runs for a period of time, the $n$ nodes are assigned into $m$ communities according to the probability of visiting different communities. In this model, the number of $m$ and $n$ are variables which can be assigned by users, and any node maybe belongs to different community in different periods. Hence this network model is time-varying. The CMOT includes two parts: intra-community forwarding and inter-community transmission. The former adopts multi-copy forwarding strategy according to the counter probability between nodes within a community, while the latter selects optimal path between the connected communities according to nodes' transmission probability. As this scheme considers both local community characteristic and the connectivity among communities in global network, it would be feasible to achieve the optimal performance. Our major contributions are summarized as following:

- We define a community-based mobile network model, and periodically compute the visiting community probability vector for each node. Then we assign the community label to each node according to the highest probability in each visiting community probability vector. This method can fit time-varying mobile social network well.
- We adopt different message delivery strategies for intra-community and inter-community message delivery. These methods not only increase message successful delivery ratio, but also decrease the algorithm complexity.
- Using message opportunistic forwarding transitivity, we can calculate the transmission probability of a node to an inaccessible community, then find the optimal path to destination community.
- An ACK mechanism is introduced to eliminate redundant message copies. Using the encounter opportunity between nodes, we adopt one-hop forwarding in local community. These methods can effectively decrease network overload.

# 3   Network Model and Community Division

## 3.1   Network Model

In this section, we define a community-based mobile network model as follows:

**Definition 1** *Network Model*: Assume that a network has $n$ nodes which can be divided by $m$ communities. The network model is expressed with $G = \{C, P\}$, where $C = \{c_i | c_i \in C, 1 \leq i \leq m\}$ is the set of communities, and $P = \{P_j | P_j \in P, 1 \leq j \leq n\}$ is the set of probability vector that a node visits each community. $P_j$ is a $m$-dimensional probability vector.

**Definition 2** *Local Community*: The community which the nodes belong to is called the local community.

**Definition 3** *Accessible Community*: The community which a node can visit is called the accessible community for this node. Obviously, the local community is one of accessible communities for a node.

**Definition 4** *Inaccessible Community*: The community which a node can not visit is called the inaccessible community for this node. A community is an accessible community for some nodes, and it can be an inaccessible community for other nodes.

**Definition 5** *Community Activity*: The community activity presents the agglomeration degree of community. When a community owns high activity, the nodes in the local community will get a large probability to go to other communities.

   To facilitate the description and analysis, the mobility model of nodes is assigned following assumptions:

- In a period, each node belongs to only one community, and nodes move in the local community for most of the time. Nodes mobility within a community follows Random-Waypoint mobility model.
- When a node leaves the local community, it will select an accessible community at random, and stays for a period of time, then selects the next community. The probability that a node leaves the local community is determined by the community activity.

## 3.2 Community Division

Depending on the definitions of the network model, we periodically count the number of times that node $i$ visits each community at initialization phase. Thereby we get the probability vector of node $i$ visiting each community. The probability vector is indicated with $P_i = \langle p_{ic_1}, p_{ic_2}, \ldots, p_{ic_j}, \ldots, p_{ic_m} \rangle$. In this expression, $p_{ic_j}$ can be computed by Formula (1), where $N_{ic_j}$ indicates the number of node $i$ visiting community $j$. The community that node $i$ visits with the highest probability is the local community of node $i$. We create a community label for node $i$ and assume that nodes in the same community have the same community label. When all nodes have confirmed their community labels, the $n$ nodes are assigned into $m$ communities in MSN.

$$p_{ic_j} = \frac{N_{ic_j}}{\sum_{k=1}^{m} N_{ic_k}} \qquad (1)$$

The above method of community division owns the advantages as following:

- The community division is not manually defined, it abides by the node self movement regularity in mobile social networks.
- With the mobility of nodes, the existing community structure may change over time in the network. In this case, the number of nodes that visit each community in a period may change. The probability vector needs to be recalculated, and the community label needs to be updated again. A new network model comes into being, it can fit time-varying mobile social network well.

## 4 Message Transmission Strategies of CMOT

### 4.1 Intra-community Forwarding Strategy

PRoPHET is a classical probability-based transmission algorithm that defines the delivery predictability to measure delivery probability metric between nodes. If the delivery predictability of node $j$ is larger than that of node $i$ which carries with messages, the node $j$ can gain a copy of the messages. Since nodes move in a community frequently and the encounter probability between nodes is high, there are large number of copies in MSN. In this case, a great deal of unnecessary messages are forwarded, they waste a lot of network resources. Therefore, we propose an improved PRoPHET algorithm for intra-community message transmission in this paper. We select one-hop nodes for destination node as relay nodes. This way ensures high delivery ratio and reduce redundant message copies.

**Encounter Prediction Probability Between Nodes** Each node holds an encounter probability vector to store encounter probability between nodes. The calculation of encounter probability between nodes is divided into encounter updating and time aging. Whenever node $i$ encounters node $j$, delivery predictability should be updated according to the Formula (2), where $p_{init} \in [0, 1]$ is an initialization constant. This formula ensures that nodes have high delivery predictability when they are often encountered.

$$p_{(i,j)} = p_{(i,j)_{old}} + \left(1 - p_{(i,j)_{old}}\right) \times p_{init} \tag{2}$$

If node $i$ does not encounter node $j$ during a time interval, they are less likely to become good forwarders of messages to each other. As a consequence, the delivery predictability must age. The aging equation is shown in Formula (3), where $\gamma \in [0, 1]$ is the aging constant, and $k$ is the number of time units. The time unit can be different, and should be defined based on the average interval of nodes encounter within the community.

$$p_{(i,j)} = p_{(i,j)_{old}} \times \gamma^k \tag{3}$$

The simulation results shown in Sect. 5 reveal that $p_{init} = 0.75$ and $\gamma = 0.98$ are the most appropriate values.

**Message Forwarding Process in a Community** Intra-community message forwarding depends on the encounter prediction probability of a node. When two nodes encounter, the CMOT compares the encounter prediction probability, and the messages always forward to the node whose encounter prediction probability is larger. If a node forwards a message to another node, it does not delete the message. If a node relays a message, it stores and manages the message in accordance with the "first-in first-out" principle, until the TTL (the time to live) value expires or the message is transferred to the destination node.

Meanwhile, an ACK mechanism is introduced to eliminate redundant message copies in the network. If the messages are forwarded to the destination node, an ACK packet that carries the ID of the received message is sent to the network. When a node receives the ACK packet, it will eliminate the redundant message copies based on the ACK information.

From the perspective of energy saving, this message forwarding method selects the node with the highest encounter probability as a relaying node to ensure the reliability of delivery. And it selects only one-hop node as the relaying node to reduce the number of redundant copies in the network.

## 4.2   Inter-community Transmission Strategy

The core of inter-community message transmission is to find the optimal path from the source node community to the destination node community.

**Community Transmission Probability. Definition 6** *Community transmission probability* The probability that a message is delivered to a community is called community transmission probability. Each node holds a community transmission probability table that stores the transmission probability from the node to each community. The community transmission probability is divided into two categories: the accessible community transmission probability and the inaccessible community transmission probability. For the local community, the value of community transmission probability is 1. For the accessible community and the inaccessible community, the values of community transmission probability are calculated as following.

*Accessible Community Transmission Probability* A node can directly visit the accessible community to create a communication path between the local community and the accessible community. Therefore, the probability that a node visits the accessible community represents its transmission probability, which is shown in Formula (4).

$$p_{ic_j} = \frac{N_{ic_j}}{\sum_{c_k \in C_a} N_{ic_k}} \tag{4}$$

where $p_{ic_j}$ is the community transmission probability of node $i$ visiting community $c_j$, $C_a$ is the accessible community set of node $i$, $N_{ic_j}$ is the number which node $i$ visits community $c_j$. In general case, the number of times is updated in each mobile cycle.

*Inaccessible Community Transmission Probability* We assume that $c_x$ is the local community of node $i$, $c_y$ is the local community of node $j$ and the accessible community of node $i$, and $c_z$ is the accessible community of node $j$ and the inaccessible community of node $i$. This indicates that there are two community communicating paths: (1) $c_x \rightarrow c_y$ that is established by node $i$, and (2) $c_y \rightarrow c_z$ that is established by node $j$. The scenario is shown in Fig. 1.

If nodes $i$ and $j$ encounter each other, they exchange the community transmission probability table. A communication path from community $c_x$ to community $c_z$ (i.e. $c_x \rightarrow c_y \rightarrow c_z$) is established when node $i$ encounters node $j$, it connects the community communicating path $c_x \rightarrow c_y$ and $c_y \rightarrow c_z$. Node $i$ has an opportunity to transfer messages from $c_x$ to $c_z$ through $c_y$.

**Fig. 1** The community path
$(c_x \rightarrow c_y \rightarrow c_z)$ is built by
nodes $i$ and $j$

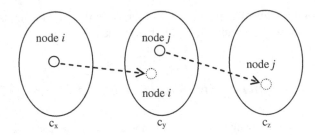

Equation (5) shows the transmission probability of node $i$ to the inaccessible community $c_z$.

$$p_{ic_z} = p_{ic_y} \times p_{(i,j)} \times p_{jc_z} \tag{5}$$

where $p_{ic_y}$ indicates the transmission probability of node $i$ to the community $c_y$, and builds the community path $c_x \rightarrow c_y$. Likewise, $p_{jc_z}$ indicates the transmission probability of node $j$ to the community $c_z$, and builds the community path $c_y \rightarrow c_z$. $p_{(i,j)}$ indicates the encounter probability of nodes $i$ node $j$, and provides the opportunity that the messages can transmit from the community $c_x$ to the community $c_z$.

Formula (5) shows that the message can transfer to the inaccessible community through the relay community. When the message delivers to a further community, it needs across more relay communities, and gets a low community transmission probability.

The node constantly updates the transmission probability of the inaccessible community during mobility. The updating operation is divided into the replacement update and the aging update.

The replacement update is described as follows: if nodes $i$ and $k$ encounter each other, a new communication path to the community $c_z$ is built. According to Formula (5), we can calculate the community transmission probability $p_{ic_z}^{new}$. Comparing $p_{ic_z}^{new}$ with the old value of the transmission probability $p_{ic_z}^{old}$, if $p_{ic_z}^{new} > p_{ic_z}^{old}$, the new value will update the old value in the community transmission probability table.

On the other side, the communication path from the source community to the destination community maybe has multiple paths. These paths dynamically change as time goes on. If the transmission probability is not updated for a period of time, it should age. The giving process is shown as Formula (6):

$$p_{ic_z}^{new} = p_{ic_z}^{old} * \eta^T \tag{6}$$

where $\eta \in [0, 1]$ is an initialized constant. The simulation results show that $\eta = 0.98$ is an ideal constant value. $T$ is the number of time unit. The time unit is variable, it is defined with the transmission delay expectation that the node moves among different communities.

**Inter-Community Message Forward Process** When messages are forwarded between communities, the transmission probability of a node to the target communities is used to choose the best community communication path. Thus, the node with the highest transmission probability is often chosen as a forwarding node between communities, until the message is delivered to the target communities.

# 5 Simulations Scenario and Results

## 5.1 Simulation Scenario and Parameters

In this paper, we use the ONE (Opportunistic Network Environment) to simulate, and compare with typical algorithms such as PRoPHET, Spray and Wait, MaxProp and CMTS. Communities are laid out as $4 \times 4$. The boundary for each community is set as a circle with a fixed center and a variable radius. Before the simulation begins, the pretreatment process of 10,000 s completes the community division. The specific simulation parameters are set in Table 1.

**Table 1** The parameters of simulation scenario

| Category | Parameter (unit) | Values |
|---|---|---|
| Scenario features | Simulation time (s) | 60,000 |
| | Simulation region (m²) | 7500 m × 7500 m |
| Community characteristics | Community quantity | 16 |
| | Community distribution | 4 × 4 |
| | The radius of community (m) | 100/300/500/700/900 |
| | The number of nodes in a community | 10 |
| Node characteristics | Mobility model | Random waypoint |
| | Movement speed (m/s) | 0–7 |
| | Community activity | 0.03/0.06/0.09/0.12/0.15/0.18/0.21 |
| | Transmission rate (KB/s) | 250 |
| | The maximum transmission range (m) | 30 |
| | Cache size (MB) | 10 |
| | Wait time (s) | 5–10 |
| Data packet characteristics | Event generator | External events |
| | Data packet size (MB) | 0.5–1.5 |
| | TTL (s) | 1000/2000/4000/6000/8000/12000 |
| | The total number of data packets | 1000 |

## 5.2   Experimental Results and Analysis

Based on the above scenario, we compare the performance of five algorithms with different parameters for community size, community activity, nodes average speed, and messages TTL. The metrics include (1) the average delay, (2) the average hops, (3) the overhead ratio, and (4) the successful delivery ratio.

**The Impact of Community Size**   The simulation results are shown in Figs. 2 and 3. The successful delivery ratio and average hops decrease when the radius size of community increase, and all algorithms have the same trends. Compared with the other four algorithms, the delivery ratio and average hops of CMOT both increase by 5–30 %. Especially when the community radius is less than 500 m, the CMOT owns higher delivery ratio than other four algorithms. This situation shows that CMOT is more suitable for small community sizes in MSNs.

The overhead ratio defined as Formula (7), indicates the communication costs in the mobile social network when messages are delivered successfully.

$$overhead\_ratio = \frac{relayed - deliveried}{deliveried} \qquad (7)$$

In Fig. 3, we can see that the COMT has somewhat higher overhead ratio than others, but it gets the worst average delay. Since the COMT has high delivery ratio and average hops, messages need to cross more communities to arrive at the destination node and take more time to finish delivery process than other algorithms.

**The Impact of Community Activity**   As shown in Fig. 4, when the community activity increases, the delivery ratio improves, while the average hops rarely change. In addition, the CMOT shows the best delivery ratio and average hops among all methods. Figure 5 shows that the overhead ratio reduces when the community activity increases, while average delay increased slowly. The COMT shows better overhead ratio than PRoPHET, MaxProp, CMTS, but it gets a higher

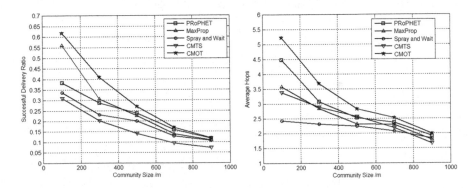

**Fig. 2**   Comparison of delivery ratio and average hops in different community sizes

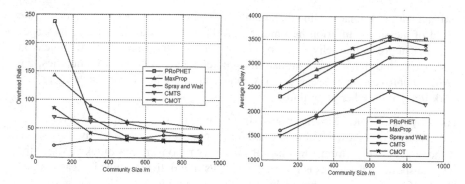

**Fig. 3** Comparison of overhead ratio and average delay in different community sizes

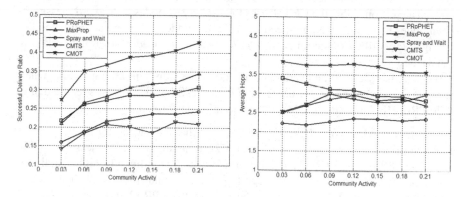

**Fig. 4** Comparison of delivery ratio and average hops in different community activity

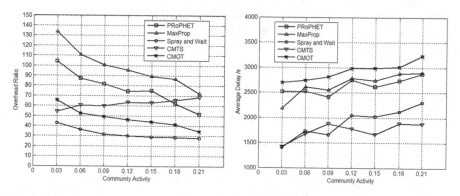

**Fig. 5** Comparison of overhead ratio and average delay in different community activity

overhead ratio than the Spray and Wait. However, the CMOT has the longest average delay in all algorithms. Although the CMTS uses community character-istics of nodes, the active node can only carry a copy to an accessible community and can not get to inaccessible communities. When the node activity increases, the speed of messages diffusion becomes faster. This increased diffusion of messages does not improve the delivery ratio, but it increases the network communication load. Using the transmission probability prediction for nodes to communities, the CMOT improves the message delivery ratio. But the CMOT consumes more network delay than other algorithms.

**The Impact of Node Moving Speed** In Fig. 6, we can see that the delivery ratio and average hops show the similar trend for all algorithms. When the average speed of the nodes changes from 1 to 4 m/s, the delivery ratio increases quickly. When the average speed of the nodes is greater than 4 m/s, the delivery ratios increase rarely. The CMOT shows the highest delivery ratio, comparing with other methods.

Figure 7 shows that the overhead ratio of CMOT increases slowly when the average speed of nodes increases, while the other algorithms have opposite tendency. The reason is that the CMOT uses the activity of nodes to forward messages. When nodes have high average speed in MSN, the nodes own high activity, and the messages forwarding opportunity increases, so the overhead ratio in network gets high value.

We can also see that the average delays decrease slowly in all algorithms when the average speed of nodes increases. And the CMTS has the lowest average delay, while PRoPHET, MaxProp, CMOT have similar performance.

**The Impact of Messages' TTL** Figure 8 shows that the successful delivery ratios of all algorithms are low when the message TTL is small. When the message TTL is higher than 4000 s, the CMOT algorithm achieves a significantly higher delivery ratio than other algorithms. The average hops have similar trend as well. Figure 9 shows that the CMOT has lower overhead ratio than PRoPHET, MaxProp, and CMTS, but has a little higher overhead ratio than the Spray and Wait. For whole time, overhead ratio curve of CMOT is smooth. This indicates that CMOT algorithm is not sensitive to the change of message TTL. The average delays increase for all algorithms when the message TTL increases, and the CMOT has longer average delay than other methods.

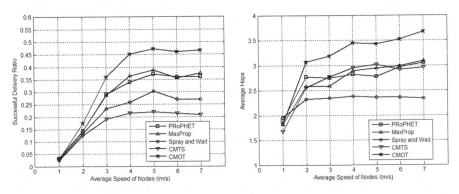

**Fig. 6** Comparison of delivery ratio and average hops in different nodes' average speed

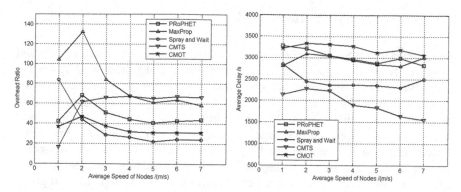

**Fig. 7** Comparison of overhead ratio and average delay in different nodes' average speed

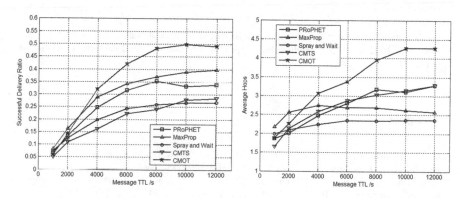

**Fig. 8** Comparison of delivery ratio and average hops in different TTL

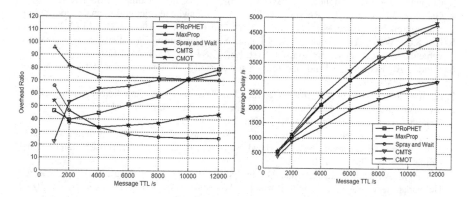

**Fig. 9** Comparison of overhead ratio and average delay in different TTL

# 6 Conclusion and Future Work

We modeled an MSN into a time-varying community-based network, and proposed a community-aware message opportunistic transmission algorithm (CMOT) in this paper. We divided the CMOT algorithm into two parts: (1) for inter-community messages transmission, the CMOT chooses an optimal community path by comparing the community transmission probability, (2) for intra-community in local community, messages are forwarded according to the encounter probability between nodes. Meanwhile we used an ACK mechanism to eliminate redundant message copies, and adopt one-hop opportunistic forwarding between nodes in intra-community to decrease network communication load. Compared with previous classical routing algorithms, the CMOT achieves the optimal performance in the message delivery ratio and overhead ratio, but the average delay is longer than that of others.

**Acknowledgment** This work is partially supported by the National Natural Science Foundation of China (61162002, 61364023), and the Jiangxi province National Natural Science Foundation of China (20151BAB207038).

# References

1. Cerf, V., Burleigh, S., Hooke, A., Torgerson, L., Durst, R., Scott, K., et al.: Delay-tolerant networking architecture. Heise Zeitschriften Verlag (2007)
2. Wu, J., Xiao, M., Huang, L.: Homing spread: community home-based multi-copy routing in mobile social networks. In: INFOCOM, 2013 Proceedings IEEE, pp. 2319–2327 (2013)
3. Ma, C., Yang, J., Du, Z., Zhang, C.: Overview of routing algorithm in pocket switched networks. In: 9th International Conference on Broadband and Wireless Computing, Communication and Applications (BWCCA), pp. 42–46. IEEE Computer Society (2014)
4. Gaito, S., Maggiorini, D., Rossi, G.P., Sala, A.: Bus switched networks: an ad hoc mobile platform enabling urban-wide communications. Ad Hoc Netw. **10**(6), 931–945 (2012)
5. Hu, S.C., Wang, Y.C., Huang, C.Y., Tseng, Y.C.: Measuring air quality in city areas by vehicular wireless sensor networks. J. Syst. Softw. **84**(11), 2005–2012 (2011)
6. Vahdat, A., Becker, D.: Epidemic routing for partially-connected ad hoc networks. Master Thesis (2000)
7. Spyropoulos, T., Psounis, K., Raghavendra, C.S.: Spray and wait: an efficient routing scheme for intermittently connected mobile networks. In: Proceedings of ACM Workshop on Delay-tolerant Networking (WDTN) (2005)
8. Spyropoulos, T., Psounis, K., Raghavendra, C.S.: Spray and focus: efficient mobility-assisted routing for heterogeneous and correlated mobility. In: Fifth Annual IEEE International Conference, pp. 79–85. IEEE (2007)
9. Lindgren, A., Doria, A., Schelén, O.: Probabilistic Routing in Intermittently Connected Networks. Service Assurance with Partial and Intermittent Resources. Springer, Berlin (2004)
10. Burgess, J., Gallagher, B., Jensen, D., Levine, B.N.: MaxProp: routing for vehicle-based disruption-tolerant networks. In: 25th IEEE International Conference on Computer Communications, pp. 1–11. IEEE (2006)
11. Niu, J., Zhou, X., Liu, Y., Sun, L.: A message transmission scheme for community-based opportunistic network. J Comput. Res. Dev. **46**(12), 2068–2075 (2009)

12. Hui, P., Crowcroft, J.: How small labels create big improvements. In: Proceedings of IEEE Percom Workshop on Intermittently Connected Mobile Ad Hoc Networks, pp. 65–70 (2007)
13. Hui, P., Crowcroft, J., Yoneki, E.: Bubble rap: social-based forwarding in delay-tolerant networks. IEEE Trans. Mob. Comput. **10**(11), 1576–1589 (2010)
14. Xiao, M., Wu, J., Huang, L.: Community-aware opportunistic routing in mobile social networks. Comput. IEEE Trans. **63**(7), 1682–1695 (2014)
15. Zhu, Y.: Social and location based routing in delay tolerant networks. Dissertations and Theses —Gradworks (2013)
16. Bulut, E., Szymanski, B.K.: Friendship based routing in delay tolerant mobile social networks. In: IEEE Global Telecommunications Conference, pp. 1–5. IEEE (2010)

# Educational Artefacts as a Foundation for Development of Remote Speech-Language Therapies

Tihomir Orehovački, Dijana Plantak Vukovac
and Tatjana Novosel-Herceg

**Abstract** Telehealth refers to the delivery of health care services at a distance by the use of information and communication technologies (ICT). Due to numerous advantages such as the enhancement of the treatment or reaching remotely located people who need treatment at affordable cost, telehealth is nowadays widely used in speech-language pathology (SLP) services. This paper presents the results of two empirical studies carried out among SLP stakeholders. The objective of the first study was to determine the state-of-the-art in using ICT among speech-language professionals and their clients in Croatia. The objective of the second study was to examine content validity and relevance of the introduced set of attributes meant for evaluating quality of educational artefacts employed in SLP therapies. Findings of both studies can be employed as a foundation for the design and implementation of the telerehabilitation systems aimed to assist in the delivery of remote speech-language therapies.

**Keywords** Speech-Language pathology · Telehealth · eHealth · Telerehabilitation

A prior version of this paper has been published in the ISD2015 Proceedings (http://aisel.aisnet.org/isd2014/proceedings2015/).

T. Orehovački (✉)
Department of Information and Communication Technologies,
Juraj Dobrila University of Pula, Pula, Croatia
e-mail: tihomir.orehovacki@unipu.hr

D. Plantak Vukovac
Faculty of Organization and Informatics, University of Zagreb,
Varaždin, Croatia
e-mail: dijana.plantak@foi.hr

T. Novosel-Herceg
VaLMod Speech-Language Pathology Centre, Varaždin, Croatia
e-mail: tatjana.novoselherceg@gmail.com

# 1    Introduction

eHealth is a broad term, also known as telehealth, that encompasses many areas that deal with health care at a distance by using ICT. While it includes domains such as telemedicine, "telehealth encompasses a variety of health care and health promotion activities, including, but not limited to, education, advice, reminders, interventions, and monitoring of interventions" [1]. Interventions such as delivery of therapeutic rehabilitation services at a distance by using modern information-communication technologies are becoming more common in physical therapy, neuropsychology, speech-language pathology and other areas.

Speech-language pathology (SLP) has been a leading profession in the use of telerehabilitation since the 1970s, by employing a telephone and mailed printed materials [2]. Today, SLP benefits a lot from recent advancements in ICT, e.g. it provides equitable access to SLP services and reduction of service costs [2], thus improving the quality of care and the quality of life of people who need these kinds of services.

Technologies used in SLP telepractice can range from the simple ones, such as e-mail or photos that are exchanged between an SLP professional and a client, to the more complex ones, like the use of videoconferencing systems for real-time communication or expert systems for diagnostic assessment. Therapists can use a myriad of ICT tools for SLP telerehabilitation, depending on the specific environment and user population. Some technologies and applications are useful for SLP professionals to enhance their everyday work and the rehabilitation process, and some online services are beneficial for the SLP clients' rehabilitation process. In that respect, the development of applications and systems in this specific field will depend on users' computer literacy and their needs.

In order to provide a better insight into speech-language pathology telehealth services offered in Croatia, two empirical studies have been carried out. The objective of the first one was to reveal the current state of the practice in use of ICT and digital services among SLP professionals and their clients [3]. Professionals and clients' needs as well as their preferences in delivering telehealth services have been elicited for that purpose. The objective of the second study was to explore content validity and relevance levels of the initial pool of attributes suggested for measuring the quality of educational artefacts. Findings presented in this paper can be employed as a foundation for development and implementation of telerehabilitation systems aimed to assist in the delivery of remote speech-language therapies.

The remainder of the paper is structured as follows: the second section provides brief literature review of characteristics of telehealth in speech-language pathology. The results of two empirical studies are presented in the third section. The implications for researchers and practitioners are discussed in the last section.

# 2 Telehealth in SLP

## 2.1 Features of Telehealth/Telerehabilitation in SLP

The main characteristic of many speech and language therapies is that they require continuous work of the SLP therapist and the client during several weeks or months, both in SLP office and at client's home. Many treatments received in the therapists' offices are usually followed by homework that patients have to practice until the next visit to the therapist. Even when the official treatment of the patients' disorders is already over, some disorders like stuttering require a continuum of supervision. Frequent visits to SLP therapists present substantial costs to the patient (or his/her family) as well as to the healthcare system. This can be easily reduced with the employment of the Internet and sophisticated technologies to provide rehabilitation at a distance.

On the other hand, SLP therapist is not always accessible to patients, e.g. to those who live in rural or distant areas or to those whose mobility is limited due to their health condition. Since the population of our society is aging, it is likely that more chronic disabilities will occur, which will reduce the capacity to move easily [2]. It is therefore necessary to come up with new ways of delivering SLP services by means of ICT, in order to improve the quality of healthcare.

In general, telerehabilitation enables SLP to optimize timing, intensity and sequencing of intervention [4], provide sustained intervention, and facilitate self-management [2].

Croatian SLP telehealth still lags behind current trends in the developed countries, but nevertheless, computer-aided speech and language therapy is present in almost every SLP office. Some institutions use specific hardware and software for rehabilitation of a particular disorder as presented in [3]. In the past two years, there have been more research and practical implementation of research results in the area of SLP telerehabilitation. Under the umbrella of the EU-funded project ICT-AAC (*ICT Competence Network for Innovative Services for Persons with Complex Communication Needs*), innovative Web applications and mobile applications for Android and iOS have been developed, targeted for persons with complex communication needs. The main feature of the applications is that they provide augmentative and alternative communication to target group to be able to respond to everyday communicative challenges [5].

In recent years, there has been an increasing interest among SLP professionals in the use of advanced ICTs in order to provide online SLP practice. More and more SLP institutions employ Internet technologies and applications to enhance their services and enable continuity of re/habilitation. The main example of this trend is the use of e-mail and smartphones to enable faster scheduling and more frequent contacts between the client and the speech therapist for the purpose of the therapy supervision and keeping it on a high-quality level. However, prior to this study, there was little evidence about the use and perceptions on SLP telerehabilitation in Croatia.

## 2.2   ICT for SLP Services

ICT can tremendously enhance SLP practice and enable accessibility of SLP services to more people in need. There is a wide range of technologies that can be used to support SLP telepractice.

ASHA, *the American Speech-Language-Hearing Association,* identifies three types of ICTs used in telepractice [6]:

- synchronous technologies for real-time audio and video interaction (e.g. telephone, audio and videoconferencing systems),
- asynchronous technologies for capturing and transmitting clinical data (e.g. capturing photos, recording voice and video, storing audio and video clips, receiving and storing users assignments by e-mail or other services and systems, etc.), and
- hybrid technologies as a combination of two aforementioned technologies.

Technologies are supported by various types of applications and information systems, which can be categorized into three working areas of SLPs:

- *ICT for SLP assessment and diagnosis*: online collaboration environments [7], and expert systems [8];
- *ICT for SLP therapies*: special software applications [9, 10], game applications [9], communication software like Skype [11], media editing software like Audacity [11], e-learning systems [12], mobile applications [5, 13];
- *ICT for the management of SLP practice*: Web information services (specialized Websites for SLP professionals and SLP clients; forums, social networks), Web services for the education and training of SLP professionals, systems for logging clients' records, systems for storing SLPs documentation (e.g. informed consent, feedback, surveys), administration of therapies, reimbursement, therapy scheduling [14].

The choice of technologies that should be used in SLP telepractice largely depends on the client population being served, the cost of equipment, available training and technology support, the level of network connectivity [2], as well as on the clients' computer and information literacy.

## 3   Results

### 3.1   First Study

**Methodology**. Considering advancements in SLP services presented in the previous sections, the authors of this paper conducted a research in July and August 2013, in order to identify state-of-the-practice in the use of ICT between two categories of SLP users in Croatia: speech-language professionals and their clients.

The research had two goals: (1) to reveal frequency of using ICT among SLP users and their computer literacy, and (2) to identify users' needs regarding SLP therapies provided online.

The research was administered as a Web questionnaire, which had two branches: one with the questions adapted to the SLP professionals and the other adapted to the SLP clients. Having in mind that many SLP clients are children, questions were formed in such a manner that parents can provide answers for their minors. Ethical issues such as voluntary participation, anonymity and data confidentiality were taken into consideration while preparing the questionnaire and inviting the users to participate in the research, as well as during the analysis of the gathered data.

A research sample for both user categories was compiled using non-probability snowball sampling which is appropriate for locating members of a specific population. An invitation to participate in a survey was distributed by e-mail to speech-language therapists using the distribution list of the Croatian Logopedic Association that had about 450 members at the time the research was taking place. SLP clients were recruited by posting an invitation to several forums dedicated to SLP topics. In order to reach a greater client population, a printed version of the Web questionnaire was also distributed to the patients of the Speech and Hearing Department of the General Hospital Varaždin. Although this might have introduced additional bias to the sample, this decision was made because many clients of the aforementioned department arrive from different parts of Croatia and even abroad. Data gathered from SLP professionals and SLP clients was analyzed with SPSS tool version 19. The following section provides preliminary analyses of data using descriptive statistics.

**Findings related to SLP Professionals** Thirty-six SLP professionals, one male and others female, completed the questionnaire. The majority of them (55.6 %) were SLP therapists from the City of Zagreb. They provided SLP therapies in the following settings: preschool (44 %), healthcare (22.2 %), school (19.4 %), social welfare institution (5.6 %), private SLP office (5.6 %), and an assistant in tertiary education (2.8 %).

A. *Use of ICT and Computer Literacy among SLP professionals*

The use of ICT and the level of computer literacy were investigated with several questions. First, the authors of this paper wanted to determine the frequency of computer usage and the Internet usage in their professional life. According to participants' responses, computers are not used to a large extent in Croatian SLP practices. Most of SLP professionals (38.9 %) use the computer for up to two hours during their working hours. Many of them use it for less than one hour (30.6 %). The minority of SLP professionals use the computer for up to three hours or more (13.9 % for both categories). One respondent (school SLP therapist) indicated that she does not have a computer at her workplace. A significant number of SLP professionals (11.1 %) do not have Internet access at work; however, most of them (66.7 %) use the Internet on a daily basis.

Study participants revealed that they use different kinds of ICT equipment for work, but the use of desktop computers prevails (77.8 %). Other equipment, like tablets or smartphones, is much less used. Even standard SLP equipment, like headphones or microphones, is not used to a large extent. Four respondents mentioned the employment of a special digital SLP set that can be used without the computer and one respondent uses a biofeedback device in her SLP practice.

Study participants who have Internet access use it for various activities to enhance their service as well as to educate themselves. SLP professionals mostly use e-mail communication with their clients, whereas file sharing or synchronous communication are used sparingly. More results on the use of ICT among SLP professionals are presented in [3].

B. *SLP professionals' needs and preferences regarding SLP therapies provided online*

In the second part of the questionnaire, SLP professionals expressed their attitudes towards employing remote speech-language therapies as well as preferences regarding type of activities they would like to apply.

Almost 70 % of study participants expressed their readiness to provide SLP therapies online. Most of them are interested to do that only periodically (61.1 %), while two of them (8.3 %) would like to provide online therapies most of the time. The majority of speech therapists who declined willingness to do online treatments were preschool therapists. One might speculate that their answer is connected with the specificities of the treatments that involve children, like security and ethical issues, correctness of the therapy performance, etc.

A vast majority of study participants (68.0 %) were willing to provide online therapies not only during official treatments but also after the treatment is over, by providing periodical online supervision of the patients. However, SLP therapists estimated that their clients are not very interested to participate in remote speech-language therapies: 68 % of therapists think that only up to 20 % of their current clients would like to participate in online therapies, while 20 % of SLP therapists estimated the percentage of interested clients to be between 20 and 40 %.

SLP professionals also revealed the amount of time they would like to be engaged in the implementation of SLP therapy sessions remotely. Compared to the time used for conventional face-to-face therapies, the majority of SLP professionals (48 %) would like to spend less time providing online therapies, while 44 % of them would spend approximately the same amount of time for online therapies as for face-to-face therapies. Only two respondents (8 %) expressed willingness to spend up to 20 % more time than in face-to-face therapies.

Online activities that SLP professionals (N = 25) would like to perform during treatment are presented in Table 1.

Almost all activities enlisted in Table 1 are considered highly acceptable apart from communication via messages or audio link. The reason for that might lie in the fact that those two activities are already incorporated into SLP practice, e.g. speaking exercise on the phone or texting on the mobile phone to agree on the schedule.

**Table 1** Preferred activities to be used in online SLP practice

| Type of preferred activity | % |
|---|---|
| Providing homework (tasks) to the patient until the next session with the therapist | 96.0 |
| Having a possibility to create their own assessment or rehabilitation content | 84.0 |
| Communicating with the patient/parent via video link | 80.0 |
| Using questionnaires for the assessment of disorders | 76.0 |
| Providing a particular therapy as a video demonstration | 76.0 |
| Providing a particular therapy as a video game | 72.0 |
| Providing constant online monitoring of the progress of a patient on treatment | 72.0 |
| Management of electronic patient record | 72.0 |
| Communicating with the patient/parent via instant messages | 48.0 |
| Communicating with the patient/parent via audio link | 36.0 |

Enlisted activities can be regarded as user needs that could be translated to user requirements during the development of SLP telerehabilitation system that would provide three main functionalities: patient's records management, SLP disorder assessments and SLP therapies. Given that continuance of the treatment is necessary for successful rehabilitation, it is not surprising that almost all respondents would like to assign homework (a task or exercise accessed online) that patients need to perform until the next face-to-face session. In that respect, a functionality that enables tracing patients' activities or a functionality of uploading homework (e.g. scanned handwriting or audio file with pronunciation) are on the top of functional specifications for the development of SLP telerehabilitation system.

Having control over the creation of assessment or rehabilitation content is also high on the list of SLP therapists' preferred activities. Since many therapists apply their own methods in the treatment of particular disorders, this means that system solutions used in telerehabilitation should be adaptive and should provide easy content creation and content management. Video therapy is an important requirement, whether used in synchronous communication or as a video demonstration that shows the patients how to execute the rehabilitation exercise. Therefore, integrating a Web camera into the system is also an important functionality. Video games, particularly educational ones, present a type of therapy that can be easily used with children or with patients that have cognitive disorders. They are usually used as a stand-alone application (mobile or Web), so their integration into the system with the functionality of score tracking would enable monitoring of the patient's progress over the time and assist the therapist in prescribing additional therapies in order to achieve desired rehabilitation outcome.

**Findings related to SLP Clients** A total of 136 persons who use SLP services took part in the study. The majority of them (86 %) completed paper-based questionnaire whereas the remaining 14 % completed a Web-based questionnaire. Forty-eight respondents (35.3 %) were parents of children that were attending SLP therapies and eighty-eight respondents (64.7 %) were end-users of SLP therapies, 44.3 % of whom were high school students, 35.2 % were adults and 20.45 % were primary school students. Regarding gender, 85.4 % of mothers and 14.6 % of fathers in contrast to 23.9 % female end-users and 76.1 % male end-users participated in the survey.

Respondents were from 19 out of 21 Croatian counties. The majority of respondents were from The City of Zagreb county, the capital city of Croatia (twenty-three respondents or 16.9 %) while other counties were represented with between one and nine respondents. This gives a roughly uniform distribution of respondents across Croatia. Respondents from the countries in the region also completed the questionnaire: Bosnia and Hercegovina (ten respondents), Serbia (three respondents) and Austria (three respondents).

## A. *Use of ICT and Computer Literacy of SLP clients*

At the time the study was carried out, all but one respondent had a computer in their household and all of them had Internet access. This is a very optimistic result given that percentage of households with computers in Croatia was 66.3 % while Internet penetration was 64.4 % in 2013 [15], showing a slight decrease in both categories in comparison to the previous year. The timespan of computer use at home is rather high: most of the users (35.3 %) stated they use the computer for up to two hours per day, while the next major category with 30.1 % of respondents use the computer for less than an hour per day. More than 60 % of users access the Internet every day, while 20.6 % access it almost every day or one-to-three times per week (15.4 %).

Regarding the use of various information and communication technologies, respondents could have selected up to nine types of technologies in the questionnaire and add additional technology if used. The majority of respondents claimed they possessed a desktop computer in the household, while a smartphone and a laptop are the next two ICT categories that are most frequently used by study participants. Comparing this result to the one of SLP professionals, it is notable that SLP clients use smartphones to a greater extent (58.1 %) than SLP service providers (16.7 %).

Relatively low employment of peripherals like Web camera and microphone might suggest that these are not used as a stand-alone piece of equipment but as an integrated part of the laptop, smartphone, or tablet. These two, including the headphones (40.4 %) or a headset instead of the headphones and microphone are prerequisites for synchronous communication between SLP professional and the client in an online environment.

One of the activities that a sample of clients uses more than SLP professionals are services for synchronous communication like Skype (44.9 and 11.1 %, respectively), which might suggest that clients are more prone to use modern communication technologies than their therapists. The use of various Internet services by SLP clients is further presented in [3].

## B. *Needs and preferences of SLP clients regarding SLP therapies provided online*

In the second part of the questionnaire, SLP clients indicated their own or their children's disorder profiles and expressed attitudes and preferences towards employing remote speech-language therapies from their homes.

77.2 % of study participants indicated stuttering as the main reason for visiting the speech therapist. Other disorders were dyslalia (7.4 %), autism spectrum disorders (6.6 %), delayed speech development (3.7 %), dyslexia and/or dysgraphia (3.7 %), unspecified disorders of speech and language development (0.7 %) and anxiety (0.7 %).

Most of the participants (67.6 %) responded that their SLP therapists were not resident in their home county. In addition, five respondents (3.7 %) indicated that they were visiting two or more SLP therapists, one of whom is outside their hometown or county. Only 18.4 % respondents attended SLP sessions in their hometown and additional 10.3 % respondents were visiting an SLP therapist who is resident in another town of their county. These responses imply that more than 80 % of SLP clients have higher traveling costs to attend SLP sessions than those who visit SLP therapists in their hometown, and these clients are potential users of online therapies.

Indeed, more than 86 % respondents expressed their readiness to participate in online SLP sessions, 59.6 % of whom were interested to participate in it from time to time, while 27.2 % respondents were interested to participate in it most of the time. However, the respondents who selected "No" for online therapies indicated their preferences regarding the use of online SLP services later in the questionnaire.

Although a higher number of SLP clients than therapists (86.5 and 69.4 % respectively) were interested in remote online therapies, it was further explored if there is a significant difference among them. Differences between study participants (SLP therapists, parents and patients) in terms of their attitude towards employing remote speech therapies were explored with Kruskal-Wallis H statistics. The reason why this non-parametric alternative to the one-way ANOVA was applied, is because the results of Shapiro-Wilk Tests uncovered that variables involved in a pairwise comparison violate the assumption of normality in data ($p < 0.05$). Considering the set forth, the results reported in Table 2 are expressed as median values.

The analysis of the collected data revealed that there are no statistically significant differences ($H(2) = 1.420$, $p = 0.492$) between the three groups of study participants in terms of their willingness to adopt remote speech-language therapies.

The majority of SLP clients (61 %) are interested to use remote SLP services after the official treatment and they would like to use it both with the therapist's supervision and independently. More than 50 % of respondents chose remote usage during official SLP treatment: 22.1 % would use it only with the therapist's supervision and 31.6 % would use it both with and without the therapist's supervision. Only 12.5 % of study participants indicated they would prefer to use online SLP services without the therapist's supervision when the official SLP treatment is

**Table 2** Results of the Kruskal-Wallis test

| Groups of study participants | N | Mean rank | H | p |
|---|---|---|---|---|
| Speech therapists | 36 | 90.35 | 1.420 | 0.492 |
| Parents | 88 | 88.34 | | |
| Patients | 48 | 80.25 | | |
| Total | 172 | | | |

over. These results indicate that clients are aware of the importance of supervised online therapies as well as the importance to continue with exercises in a prolonged period of time.

Online activities that SLP clients ($N = 136$) would like to perform are as follows, starting with the most preferred activities: communicating with the SLP therapists via video link (68.4 %), video demonstration of a particular therapy or exercise (63.2 %), communicating with SLP therapists via audio link (33.8 %), particular therapy in the form of a video game accessed through the Web (33.8 %) and particular therapy in the form of a video game installed on a mobile phone or tablet (29.4 %).

Similar to the SLP professionals, clients considered video to be an important feature of online SLP treatments, both for communication, demonstration of exercises and improving skills using a video game.

## 3.2   Second Study

**Methodology**. The second study was carried out with two main objectives: (a) to identify a set of attributes that contribute to the quality of educational artefacts employed in speech-language therapies and (b) to determine the relevance of each quality attribute from the perspective of SLP professionals. Based on the recent advances in the field of measuring quality of Web 2.0 applications [16] and quality of educational artefacts created with the use of social web applications [17], an initial pool of twenty attributes meant for measuring diverse dimensions of quality in the context of educational artefacts used for SLP purposes was generated. Content validity of quality attributes was independently explored by SLP professionals on a three-point scale (1—mandatory, 2—desired, 3—not relevant). Data collected from SLP professionals was examined with two criteria: content validity ratio (CVR) and average value of assigned relevance ($\bar{x}$)The relevance of quality attributes which have met the cut-off values of the aforementioned criteria was assigned by SLP professionals on a nine-point scale (1—low relevance, 9—extremely high relevance). Final relevance scores were estimated as an average of inputs obtained from SLP professionals.

**Participants** A total of seven SLP professionals took part in the study. All of them were female. At the time the study was conducted, they had, on average, 8.071 (SD = 7.629) years of experience in providing speech-language therapies and were working in 4 out of 21 counties in Croatia. The same number of them (28.57 %) work with preschool or school children, or have their own private practice, whereas only one of them works in a health care facility. When the use of information and communication technology is concerned, 85.71 % of them use desktop computer, 71.43 % apply notebook and digital camera, 57.14 % employ tablets, 42.86 % use smartphones, whereas 28.57 % of them apply specific speech-language equipment while providing therapies. The majority of them (57.14 %) employ computer for at least two hours a day for the purpose of their work. Finally, 71.43 % of the study participants use Internet on a daily basis for the purpose of implementing SLP activities.

**Findings** A total of seven quality attributes (consistency, timeliness, flexibility, controllability, effectiveness, efficiency, and understandability) which did not meet the threshold values of the content validity ratio (CVR = 0.99) and average value of assigned relevance ($\bar{x} \geq 2.00$) criteria [18, 19] were omitted from further analysis. The results of both content validity and relevance analysis in the context of the attributes meant for measuring quality of educational artefacts used in speech-language therapies are presented in Table 3.

Scores shown in Table 3 indicate that quality attributes can be grouped in six different relevance levels. The extent to which the content of educational artefacts is accurate and valid (correctness), the degree to which content of educational

**Table 3** Results of the content validity and relevance analysis

| Quality attributes | CVR | $\bar{x}$ | Relevance |
|---|---|---|---|
| Accessibility | 0.99 | 1.57 | 6.14 |
| Aesthetics | 0.99 | 1.29 | 7.00 |
| Attitude | 0.99 | 1.00 | 7.86 |
| Availability | 0.99 | 1.57 | 4.57 |
| Compatibility | 0.99 | 1.71 | 5.43 |
| Consistency[a] | 0.71 | 2.00 | N/A |
| Correctness | 0.99 | 1.00 | 8.71 |
| Coverage | 0.99 | 1.00 | 8.71 |
| Credibility | 0.99 | 1.14 | 8.00 |
| Timeliness[a] | 0.99 | 2.00 | N/A |
| Flexibility[a] | 0.14 | 2.43 | N/A |
| Controllability[a] | −0.43 | 2.71 | N/A |
| Customizability | 0.99 | 1.14 | 7.57 |
| Ease of use | 0.99 | 1.43 | 7.43 |
| Effectiveness[a] | 0.71 | 1.57 | N/A |
| Efficiency[a] | 0.14 | 1.86 | N/A |
| Error prevention | 0.99 | 1.57 | 7.29 |
| Familiarity | 0.99 | 1.43 | 6.29 |
| Continuance intention | 0.99 | 1.14 | 7.86 |
| Playfulness | 0.99 | 1.57 | 6.71 |
| Satisfaction | 0.99 | 1.29 | 7.86 |
| Understandability[a] | 0.43 | 1.57 | N/A |
| Social influence | 0.99 | 1.57 | 6.71 |
| Uniqueness | 0.99 | 1.43 | 7.00 |
| Usefulness | 0.99 | 1.14 | 8.00 |
| Trackability | 0.99 | 1.43 | 6.71 |

[a]Omitted from further analysis because they did not meet content validity criteria (CVR = 0.99; $\bar{x} \geq 2.00$)

artefacts is complete and displayed clearly (coverage), the level to which content of educational artefacts is unbiased and trustworthy (credibility), and the extent to which educational artefacts are advantageous (usefulness) are, according to SLP professionals, of extremely high relevance in the context of measuring the quality of SLP educational artefacts.

The degree of users' favourableness toward using educational artefacts in speech-language therapies (attitude), the extent to which patients are willing to employ educational artefacts for the purpose of SLP therapies on a regular basis (continuance intention), the level to which the patients are pleased with the use of educational artefacts in speech-language therapies (satisfaction), the extent to which educational artefacts are adapted to meet users' needs (customizability), the degree to which the employment of educational artefacts is free of effort (ease of use), the level to which the use of educational artefacts prevents the occurrence of patient's errors while performing SLP exercises (error prevention), the degree to which educational artefacts are visually appealing (aesthetics), and the extent to which educational artefacts are distinctive (uniqueness) are attributes that have very high influence on the quality of educational artefacts.

The level to which educational artefacts are able to hold patient's attention (playfulness), the degree to which patients are motivated to use educational artefacts (social influence), the extent to which it is possible to monitor the employment of educational artefacts by patients (trackability), the level to which educational artefacts are similar to previously used SLP exercises (familiarity), and the extent to which educational artefacts can be used by people with the widest range of characteristics and capabilities (accessibility), according to results of relevance analysis, significantly contribute to the quality of educational artefacts.

The degree to which educational artefacts operate properly with different types of devices (e.g. smartphones, tablets, PCs, laptops, etc.) and among different web browsers (compatibility) together with the extent to which educational artefacts are continuously available (availability) appeared to be quality attributes with high relevance in terms of the quality of educational artefacts.

Finally, the analysis of data collected from SLP professionals revealed that attributes meant for measuring the level to which educational artefacts do not differ in their structure, design, and terminology (consistency), the degree to which educational artefacts can be modified and updated (timeliness), the extent to which patient has freedom in executing exercises (controllability), the level to which exercises can be performed accurately and completely by means of educational artefacts (effectiveness), the degree to which the use of educational artefacts improves efficiency of a patient in conducting exercises (efficiency), the extent to which educational artefacts can be employed beyond initially intended context of use (flexibility), and the level to which educational artefacts are clear and unambiguous (understandability), according to the opinion of SLP professionals, do not significantly affect the quality of educational artefacts.

# 4  Discussion and Concluding Remarks

This paper presents research results of two empirical studies conducted among Croatian SLP stakeholders: therapists and their clients. The first one was focused on the use of ICT of SLP stakeholders as well as their readiness to provide or participate in treatments conducted online. According to the responses collected in the first study, speech therapists do not use ICT to a large extent in their practice, especially modern technologies like tablets, smartphones or services for synchronous communication and file sharing with the clients. SLP patients are better equipped and more prone to use various communication services, which might be employed in the online speech-language therapies as well.

There are no statistically significant differences between the study participants in terms of their willingness to adopt remote online therapies. The first study has revealed that the majority of therapists and clients would like to use remote SLP services after the official treatment, with periodical online supervision of the clients' disorder status. Both groups of respondents indicated video as an important part of telerehabilitation, whether integrated in the systems' solution as a communication tool, a demonstration content or a game for improving skills.

The outcomes of the second study revealed content validity and relevance scores of the initial set of attributes proposed for measuring quality of educational artefacts. Although the majority of introduced attributes were perceived by SLP professionals as highly important mean for estimating quality of educational artefacts used in speech-language therapies, some of them, which proved to be essential in evaluating software quality (e.g. efficiency, effectiveness, understandability, etc.), have not been recognized as relevant by the sufficient number of SLP professionals.

Although the conducted studies have revealed some important aspects of SLP telerehabilitation that should be taken into consideration when planning and implementing systems for online therapies, the results should be taken with caution due to a few limitations in the research methodology. One of them is data collection, which was acquired using dual-mode questionnaire, with the paper version of the questionnaire taken only at one SLP institution, specialized in the treatment of stuttering. Therefore, the majority of responses were collected from the people who stutter (or their parents), so their responses might be biased and not reflecting responses of people with other speech, language, or communication disorders. Another drawback is a relatively small number of speech therapists who completed the questionnaire.

Nevertheless, the first study results indicate that SLP users in Croatia and countries in the region are aware of the benefits of remote online treatments and have met the minimum requirements in terms of ICT equipment and computer literacy to employ speech-language telerehabilitation. The findings of this study also reveal context of use and general needs of stakeholders who will use SLP telerehabilitation systems. While the first study presents a good method for the elicitation of users' needs in the early stage of system development, future work in requirements engineering for telerehabilitation systems should incorporate other methods such as interview, storytelling, and personas to refine users' needs into formal specifications. In addition, the results of the second study will be used as a backbone for modelling the interplay of the finite set of quality attributes.

**Acknowledgements** This work has been carried out within research project "eSLP—development and evaluation of the system for online SLP therapies" funded by the Adris Foundation, Croatia.

# References

1. APTA—American Physical Therapy Association. Telehealth—Definitions and Guidelines. http://www.apta.org/uploadedFiles/APTAorg/About_Us/Policies/Practice/TelehealthDefinitions Guidelines.pdf (2012). Accessed 20 Nov 2015
2. Theodoros, D.: Speech-language pathology and telerehabilitation. In: Kumar, S., Cohn, E.R. (eds.) Telerehabilitation, pp. 311–323. Springer, Heidelberg (2013)
3. Plantak Vukovac, D., Novosel-Herceg, T., Orehovački, T.: Users' needs in telehealth speech-language pathology services. In: Vogel, D., Guo, X., Barry, C., Lang, M., Linger, H., Schneider, C. (eds.) Information Systems Development: Transforming Healthcare through Information Systems (ISD2015 Proceedings). Hong Kong, SAR: Department of Information Systems. ISBN: 978-962-442-393-8. http://aisel.aisnet.org/isd2014/proceedings2015/HealthcareIS/4 (2015)
4. Winters, J.M.: Telerehabilitation interface strategies for enhancing access to health services for persons with diverse abilities and preferences. In: Kumar, S., Cohn, E.R. (eds.) Telerehabilitation, pp. 200–212. Springer, Heidelberg (2013)
5. ICT-AAC. Competence network for innovative services for persons with complex communication needs, final dissemination and visibility event. http://www.ict-aac.hr/images/news/ICT-AAC_Brosura_Zavrsni_diseminacijski_dogadjaj.pdf (2015). Accessed 20 Feb 2015
6. ASHA—American Speech-Language-Hearing Association. Telepractice. http://www.asha.org/Practice-Portal/Professional-Issues/Telepractice/ (2014). Accessed 20 Jan 2014
7. Pierrakeas, C., Georgopoulos, V., Malandraki, G.: Online collaboration environments in telemedicine applications of speech therapy. In: Proceedings of the 27th Annual International Conference of the IEEE Engineering in Medicine and Biology Society, pp. 2183–2186 (2005)
8. Toki, E.I., Pange, J., Mikropoulos, T.A.: An online expert system for diagnostic assessment procedures on young children's oral speech and language. Procedia Soc. Behav. Sci. **14**, 428–437 (2012)
9. Saz, O., Yin, S.C., Lleida, E., Rose, R., Vaquero, C., Rodríguez, W.R.: Tools and technologies for computer-aided speech and language therapy. Speech Commun. **51**(10), 948–967 (2009)
10. Toki, E.I., Pange, J.: E-learning activities for articulation in speech language therapy and learning for preschool children. In: Procedia—Social and Behavioral Sciences vol. 2, no. 2, pp. 4274–4278. Elsevier Ltd, Amsterdam (2010)
11. Carey, B., O'Brian, S., Onslow, M., Packman, A., Menzies, R.: Webcam delivery of the camperdown program for adolescents who stutter: a phase I trial. In: Nippold, M.A. (ed.) Language, Speech, and Hearing Services in Schools vol. 43, no. 3, pp. 370–380, ASHA, Rockville, USA (2012)
12. Beijer, L.J., Rietveld, T.C.M., van Beers, M.M.A., Slangen, R.M.L., van den Heuvel, H., de Swart, B.J.M., Geurts, A.C.H.: E-learning-based speech therapy: a web application for speech training. In: Telemedicine and e-Health, vol. 16, no. 2, pp. 177–180. Mary Ann Liebert, Inc., New York (2010)
13. Speech and language therapy apps, virtual speech center. https://www.virtualspeechcenter.com/MobileApps.aspx (2014). Accessed 30 Jan 2014

14. Paone, S., Shevchik, G.: Making a business case for eHealth and teleservices. In: Kumar, S., Cohn, E.R. (eds.) Telerehabilitation, pp. 297–309. Springer, Heidelberg (2013)
15. ITU. Measuring the information society report 2014. http://www.itu.int/en/ITU-D/Statistics/Pages/publications/mis2014.aspx. Accessed 30 Jan 2014
16. Orehovački, T., Granić, A., Kermek, D.: Evaluating the perceived and estimated quality in use of Web 2.0 applications. J. Syst. Softw. **86**(12), 3039–3059 (2013)
17. Orehovački, T., Žajdela Hrustek, N.: Development and validation of an instrument to measure the usability of educational artifacts created with Web 2.0 applications. In: Marcus, A. (ed.) DUXU, Part I, HCII 2013. Lecture Notes in Computer Science, vol. 8012, pp. 369–378. Springer, Las Vegas (2013)
18. Lawshe, C.H.: A quantitative approach to content validity. In: Personnel Psychology vol. 28, no. 4, pp. 563–575 (1975)
19. Lewis, J.R.: IBM computer usability satisfaction questionnaires: psychometric evaluation and instructions for use. Int. J. Hum.-Comput. Inter. **7**(1), 57–78 (1995)

# Framing or Gaming? Constructing a Study to Explore the Impact of Option Presentation on Consumers

Chris Barry, Mairéad Hogan and Ann M. Torres

**Abstract** The manner in which choice is framed influences individuals' decision-making. This research examines the impact of different decision constructs on decision-making by focusing on the more problematic decision constructs: the un-selected and pre-selected opt-out. The study employs eye-tracking with cued retrospective think-aloud (RTA) to combine quantitative and qualitative data. Eye-tracking will determine how long a user focuses on a decision construct before taking action. Cued RTA where the user will be shown a playback of their interaction will be used to explore their attitudes towards a decision construct and identify problematic designs. This pilot begins the second of a three phase study, which ultimately aims to develop a research model containing the theoretical constructs along with hypothesized causal associations between the constructs to reveal the impact of measures such as decision construct type, default value type and question framing have on the perceived value of the website and loyalty intentions.

**Keywords** Framing of choice · Decision constructs · Consumer involvement · Elaboration likelihood model · Optionality presentation · Opt-out · Must-opt · Eye-tracking

A prior version of this paper has been published in the ISD2015 Proceedings (http://aisel.aisnet.org/isd2014/proceedings2015/).

C. Barry (✉) · M. Hogan · A.M. Torres
National University of Ireland Galway, Galway, Ireland
e-mail: chris.barry@nuigalway.ie

M. Hogan
e-mail: mairead.hogan@nuigalway.ie

A.M. Torres
e-mail: ann.torres@nuigalway.ie

# 1  Introduction

This paper continues a stream of research conducted by the authors over recent years into questionable practices in the low-cost carrier (LCC) sector in Ireland and Europe. From a number of studies it was established that experts in web design and representative users found their experience to be highly problematic in fully understanding flight prices, taxes and charges, avoiding optional extras and navigating a stress-free path to a commercial conclusion. The authors found some decisions were presented to users utilizing highly unorthodox decision constructs. From here, and before conducting further planned research, a study was conducted to fully identify and compose a taxonomy of all types of decision constructs presented to users in the business-to-consumer (B2C) commercial transactional process. This paper traces the journey and lays out the formulation of a pilot study to measure how decision construct design impacts on how long it takes users to complete specific tasks. Thereafter follow several research phases to develop a framework that will enhance practitioners and researchers understanding of the impact of option presentation on the decision-making of consumers during the transactional process in B2C interactions.

# 2  Decision Framing and Gaming

## 2.1  Research on Option or Choice Framing

The framing of choice for decision-making has been the subject of research in many disciplines over the past forty years. From early classical economics, the way alternative choices were presented to decision-makers was thought not to affect an individual's capacity to rank them, assign probabilities to outcomes, and select the one with the highest utility. This rational choice model assumes an objective individual who rationally makes optimal decisions. Hence, given the same data, rational individuals would always make the same decision.

The theory of rational choice, governing social and economic behavior, has been questioned across a number of disciplines. Simon [1] was among the first to signal its limitations by proposing the concept of 'bounded rationality'. Subsequently, Tversky and Kahneman [2] theorised framed information could be encoded positively or negatively. Their research indicated the manner in which choice is framed to individuals significantly influences decision-making. They concluded the dependence of preferences on the formulation of decision problems constitutes a major concern for the theory of rational choice.

In real-world cases, Samuelson and Zeckhauser [3] found decisions are often presented with 'influential labels', whereby there is nearly always one alternative that carries the label 'status quo'. In a series of experiments designed to test for status quo effects, they concluded decision-makers exhibited a significant choice bias towards the status quo. Similarly, though in varied contexts, other studies [4–6] conclude individuals are more likely to retain a default option than to change it, even if the decision is detrimental to them. Hence, users were more likely to participate if an option is presented as an opt-out, rather than an opt-in; the reasons for which vary from: trust in a default; a presumption that it is a recommendation; and participant inertia.

Bellman et al. [4] explored the impact of question framing on user decisions. In querying how consumers have unknowingly opted-in to something, they explored the tactics some firms employ to encourage consent. They identified different ways in which consent can be obtained and concluded there are consequential effects in how questions are presented to consumers. Indeed, by using the correct combination of question framing and default answers, firms 'can almost guarantee' consent. Lai and Hui [6] also conducted research into the impact of question framing on user decisions. Their study indicates the manner in which the option is described, as well as the default option (i.e., checked or unchecked), has an impact on user choice. They found for opt-in decisions using checkboxes, users are more likely to accept an un-selected opt-in over a pre-selected opt-in. They suggest the positive language of acceptance is likely to influence the users' decision.

## 2.2 Gaming

The challenges consumers experience with online decision-making is best evidenced through the LCC industry, as it developed over the last two decades. Some carriers, such as Ryanair, promoted a brash and belligerent image to reflect that passengers were buying cheap flights and that customer service was a casualty of this Faustian pact [7].

For some LCCs, many non-sales related activities are simply removed or distanced from consumers. This deconstructed, no-frills business model is often reflected in the design of the supporting web-based information system. Conventionally, information systems seek to provide an engaging end-user experience that encourages repeat business and customer retention. However, there remains a gap between the functionality one would expect to find in sophisticated, web-based information systems and what LCCs actually offer. The route to purchase, once users pass a committal point, degenerates into an adversarial transactional process that involves consumers navigating as many as a dozen optional extras that are variously opt-in, opt-out, must-opts (see Table 1) and sometimes, repeated 'offers' suggesting consumers have not made the correct decision in rejecting the option. This practice is effectively gaming. A forgiving interpretation is that the cheap flights are enhanced by optional, ancillary charges. A more cynical interpretation is that the flight price is deconstructed into an apparent cheap headline price, but reconstructed into a much greater price via a plethora of unavoidable taxes and charges, and an array of optional charges, some of which are made difficult to avoid and are unorthodox in their design.

**Table 1** A taxonomy of decision constructs in B2C transactions

| Decision construct | Description |
|---|---|
| Un-selected opt-in | This decision construct has a default option of not receiving the option. It is generally presented as an un-ticked check box or a radio button set to off, where the option is framed in an acceptance format. Thus, the terminology states the customer wants the option |
| Pre-selected opt-in | This decision construct has a default option of not receiving the option. It is generally presented as a ticked check box or a radio button set to on, where the option is framed in a rejection format. Thus, the terminology states the customer does not want the option |
| Un-selected opt-out | This decision construct has a default option of receiving the option. It is generally presented as an un-ticked check box or a radio button set to off, where the option is framed in a rejection format. Thus, the terminology states the customer does not want the option |
| Pre-selected opt-out | This decision construct has a default option of receiving the option. It is generally presented as a ticked check box or a radio button set to on, where the option is framed in an acceptance format. Thus, the terminology states the customer wants the option |
| Must-opt | A must-opt decision occurs when an optional extra is presented to a customer as un-selected. It is not possible to proceed to the next webpage without having made a selection. It is generally presented as radio buttons, command buttons or a drop down list |
| Un-selected essential decision | An un-selected essential decision is where none of the variants has been pre-selected for the customer. Unlike the must-opt, this construct does not offer an optional extra, as the user must choose one of the presented variants. For example, the customer chooses a payment method |
| Pre-selected essential decision | A pre-selected essential decision is where one of the variants has been pre-selected for the customer. Unlike the must-opt, this construct does not offer an optional extra, as the user must choose one of the presented variants. It may be in either the customer's or the vendor's favour, or it may be neutral. For example, fast delivery for a surcharge may be pre-selected |

Due to practices by a significant number of European airlines, the European Union legally require optional extras on airline websites only be presented to consumers on an opt-in basis [8, 9]. However, Barry et al. [10], found some Irish airlines were using an unconventional design pattern to present optional extras that forced consumers to make a choice, rather than progress un-hindered. This construct, termed a 'must-opt', required users to accept or reject the item before continuing with the interaction. The study examined user perceptions of the level of compliance of two airlines with the relevant European Union legislation and found users were significantly frustrated by a long series of optional extras presented in an unorthodox manner. Neither did they believe the airlines to be compliant with the European Union requirement to communicate all optional extras in a clear, transparent and unambiguous manner. From this research, the authors went on to produce an exhaustive taxonomy of decision constructs (see Table 1) used in B2C transactional processes [11]. In testing the taxonomy, certain constructs were found to be problematic, particularly opt-outs and must-opts, in respect of the clarity of the optionality and the level of opacity [12].

The research and discussion above and in Sect. 2.1 establishes the framing and gaming of choice and the presentation of defaults have a significant impact and influence on user decision-making.

## 2.3  Involvement and the Elaboration Likelihood Model

Consumer decisions fall along a continuum of limited to extensive decision-making and it is the degree of consumer involvement that largely determines the type of decision-making [13]. Involvement reflects the amount of time and effort an individual invests in the decision-making process and is typically separated into two levels—high and low involvement. Therefore, high involvement (i.e., extensive decision-making) signals the individual cares about the decision and/or it is meaningful to them, whereas low involvement signals the opposite.

Involvement is defined as an individual's internal state, which reflects their level of arousal or interest in an object [14]. Involvement's stability makes it a key determinant of consumer behavior, as it is resistant to external influences [15]. Highly involved individuals use a more systematic process for decision-making [16]. Consequently, they exert considerable effort in searching and examining information, and carefully elaborate their beliefs with respect to a specific object [17]. In contrast, less involved individuals exhibit the opposite behavior by spending less time and engaging in fewer information seeking behaviors [18].

Relating involvement to the elaboration likelihood model (ELM), the same information can be processed in different ways, depending on the individual's level of involvement [19]. For example, individuals who are motivated (i.e., highly involved) are more likely to process a message via the central route [20]. That is, they are likely to engage in thoughtful consideration of the message and incorporate their own assessment of the arguments. Furthermore, meta-analytic research indicates that as involvement increases, so does the importance of argument quality [21].

In contrast, individuals who are unmotivated (i.e., less involved) are more likely to process a message via the peripheral routes, which represent mental shortcuts that focus on non-content cues [22]. Hence, when involvement is low, individuals are more likely to rely on peripheral cues from the stimulus (i.e., the firm). Thus, less involved consumers may simply accept what a firm recommends because they have low motivation to process content information, a similar phenomenon found in studies mentioned earlier [4–6].

Applying the ELM, one would expect individuals who spend a considerable amount of time on a decision construct are highly involved, while individuals who spend a limited amount of time on the same decision construct are less involved. The question is whether certain decision constructs (e.g., opt-outs) have the same results as those predicted with ELM. To date, no study has specifically investigated the effects of decision construct characteristics and the moderating effect of user involvement on purchasing intention. This perspective will be examined as part of the proposed research plan.

# 3  Deconstructing Options

## 3.1  Dimensions of Option Presentation

The presentation of options to consumers in contemporary B2C interactions is made up of a number of dimensions. Much of the research discussed earlier on framing largely related to a singular dimension, that of a polar decision, choosing one of two options. In the more sophisticated world of online consumerism, the presentation of choice and optionality can be greatly finessed. The presentation of an option may now have multiple, even layered, dimensions.

Previous research [11, 12] determined options tend to be presented to the user in a variety of ways. Some options are straightforward with easy to understand defaults and choices, while other options are more complicated and require effort to decipher so as to identify the default and the action required to achieve the desired outcome. In addition, some options are simply presented to the consumer while others incorporate various levels of persuasion, presumably to encourage selection of the vendor's preferred outcome. The less straightforward decision constructs encountered were pre-selected and un-selected opt-outs, must-opts and pre-selected opt-ins. This initial stage of research examines pre-selected and un-selected opt-outs while later stages will examine the other decision construct types.

A desk analysis of 57 websites was conducted to determine the fundamental dimensions of option presentation for opt-out decision constructs in use in B2C websites. A total of 42 opt-outs were encountered across 17 of the websites examined. A number of dimensions were identified as contributing to option presentation, namely:

- *control type* (e.g., check box, radio button, drop-down menu);
- *default value* (i.e., un-selected or pre-selected);
- *question or information framing* (i.e., acceptance, rejection or neutral language);
- *general purpose of the construct* (e.g., immediate revenue generation, permission to collect or retain personal data, permission to contact the consumer regarding this purchase); and
- *additional persuaders* (e.g., benefits of choosing the option, risks of rejecting the option, reassurance of privacy).

From these, the fundamental dimensions of option presentation were distilled as: default value; framing and additional persuaders. The default value is either pre-selected or un-selected. For example, a pre-selected checkbox would be pre-ticked, while an un-selected checkbox would not be ticked. The framing deals

**Table 2** Dimensions of option presentation

| Dimension | Presentation |
|---|---|
| Default value | Pre-selected or un-selected |
| Question/information framing | Acceptance, rejection or neutral |
| Additional persuaders | Yes or no |

with the way in which the question or text associated with the decision construct is presented, and can be acceptance (e.g., *Please send me the newsletter*), rejection (e.g., *I do not want travel insurance*) or neutral, where the option is simply stated (e.g., *Newsletter*). The third component of option presentation is the use of additional persuaders. The additional persuader can vary in level of persuasion from a brief statement of benefits to much more comprehensive persuaders including details on the risks associated with declining the option, extensive statement of benefits and reassurance regarding protection of privacy, security or the ability to reverse the decision if desired. The dimensions of option presentation are outlined in Table 2.

## 3.2   Exploring Opt-Out Options

Once the dimensions of option presentation were identified, the opt-outs were examined to determine how they fit in to the structure of default value, question/information framing and additional persuaders (see Table 2). Of the 42 opt-outs encountered, 36 were pre-selected and 6 were un-selected. Of the 36 pre-selected opt-outs, 26 used acceptance framing, 1 used rejection framing and 9 used neutral framing. In all cases, this neutral framing was deemed to have an acceptance slant, as the option was pre-selected. All the un-selected opt-outs used rejection framing.

The use of additional persuaders included in the decision constructs varied. Of the 26 pre-selected opt-outs that used acceptance framing, 19 used additional persuaders, including brief or extensive description of the benefits, enthusiastic language, reassurance of credibility, and detailing of the risks of declining the option. The remaining 7 used no additional persuaders. The one pre-selected opt-out using rejection framing used no additional persuaders while 6 of the 9 using neutral framing used additional persuaders and the remaining 3 did not. All 6 of the un-selected opt-outs used additional persuaders. Figure 1 summarizes these desk analysis findings.

The additional persuaders used with the opt-outs varied considerably in strength and are categorized as: none, weak, moderate or strong. A brief description of benefits was considered to be a persuader due to the positive connotations and desirability associated with terms like 'promotions' and 'special offers'. However, they would be considered weak persuaders, as they do not include extensive descriptions of the benefits (see Table 3). Moderate persuaders have more extensive detail about the benefits, or use more enthusiastic language. The use of the bold text

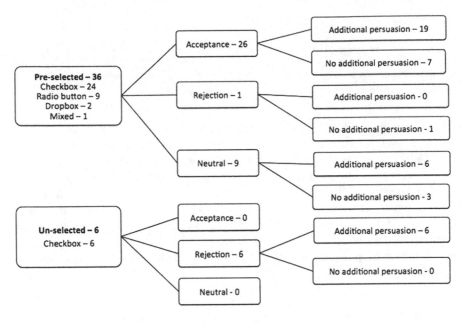

**Fig. 1** Desk analysis of option presentation in practice—opt-outs

**Table 3** Levels of persuasion

| Persuasion level | Examples |
|---|---|
| Weak | "Send me offers and promotions from ..."<br>"Please send special offers" |
| Moderate | "Sign me up! I'd like to receive promotional material from ..." |
| Strong: multiple approaches to persuade | "What if I need to cancel?<br>We understand. So, we're proud to offer cancellation insurance just in case [...] box offices don't ever allow refunds or exchanges, but since we're aware that bad weather, family emergencies and the like can arise that may prevent you from attending a show as planned you can get it from us for an additional $20.00 per ticket<br>Then we'll give you a full refund of the ticket cost (less the insurance and service fees), as long as we receive your tickets in our office at least two business days prior to the performance. Sound good?" |
| Strong: low risk in accepting option | Privacy and promotional offers<br>The privacy of our guests is our utmost concern. We will never sell or distribute your information. If you would like to receive special offers we promise to never send more than 1 email per month |

and the exclamation mark in the example in Table 3, coupled with the positive connotations associated with the term 'promotional material' would be likely to emphasize the desirability of this option.

Strong persuaders use multiple approaches to encourage the user to accept the vendor's preferred decision. Multiple examples of strong persuaders were encountered across a variety of websites. In some cases the benefits of purchase were combined with the risks of rejection. In others, the consumer was reassured that their data would be protected in addition to describing the benefits of purchase.

An example of a strong persuader was encountered when the option of cancellation insurance was presented to the consumer in the process of purchasing tickets (see Table 3). This particular example describes the risks of rejecting the option (i.e., not being able to get a refund), as well as describing the benefits of purchase (i.e., getting a refund if the consumer is unable to attend the show). It further persuades by the description of common events (e.g., bad weather) that may force the consumer to cancel and thus, reinforces the importance of purchasing insurance. Another example seeks to reassure the consumer there is little risk associated with the acceptance of the option (see Table 3). In addition to the use of the term 'special offers', which has positive connotations, this example also seeks to reassure the consumer their data will be protected and they will not receive an excessive volume of e-mails, thus minimizing the potential risks often associated with mailing lists.

# 4 Exploratory Study

## 4.1 Background to Eye-Tracking Research

Modern eye-tracking technology works on the principle of focusing a light and a video camera on a person's eye to determine where the individual is looking on screen [23]. When an individual wants to pay attention to something, they fix their gaze on it and it comes into sharp focus. This focus is referred to as a fixation. A person typically moves their eye across various items of interest. These movements, referred to as saccades, are jerky and happen so quickly, we are not aware of them. The saccades are rapid, lasting between one-hundredth and one-tenth of a second, while fixations last between one-tenth and a half second [23].

Eye-tracking has been used extensively in web usability studies [24–28]. Goh et al. [29] compared a number of usability testing techniques for an e-commerce website and found the use of *retrospective think-aloud with eye movement* (RTE) identified significantly more usability problems than *retrospective think-aloud* (RTA), observation or *feedback capture after task* (FCAT).

By studying what users do and do not look at, it is possible to determine where they are concentrating their attention [30]. Through the examination of eye movement patterns, conclusions may then be drawn on the decision-making strategies users adopt [26, 31, 32].

## 4.2   Research Plan and Approach

The research plan involves three phases [12] and is summarised in Table 4. Firstly, to identify an exhaustive list of the various decision constructs encountered when purchasing a product or service whilst on-line and then to consider some of the more salient issues that surround the transactional process. This phase, as discussed earlier, has already been conducted. Secondly, a more intense analysis, made up of two parts, of the presentation of the decision constructs, including an exploration of the juxtaposition between optionality and question framing will be conducted. Eye-tracking and cued RTA will be used as research techniques. Thirdly, a research model, broadly based on the E-S-QUAL research instrument, will be composed containing the theoretical constructs (such as service quality, social value, perceived value of website, loyalty intentions and increased peer recommendation) along with hypothesized causal associations between the constructs. Measures, unique to the study, will be validated. These will include industry category, decision construct type, default value type, persuasion and question framing.

**Table 4**   Research plan

| Phase | Description/objective | Output |
|---|---|---|
| Phase 1 | To identify an exhaustive list of decision constructs encountered in the B2C transactional process. Some of the more salient issues that surround the transactional process were examined in an exploratory analysis of 77 decision constructs from 15 websites across 5 sectors [12] | An exhaustive mutually exclusive taxonomy of all decision constructs the B2C in transactional process was constructed (see Table 1) |
| Phase 2—Part 1 | A pilot study, the subject of this paper, will be conducted to examine the impact of different decision constructs on decision-making, by focusing on the un-selected and pre-selected opt-out | It is expected the research output will validate the research design for Phase 2 |
| Phase 2—Part 2 | The results from Part 1 will inform an extensive eye-tracking and cued RTA study to comprehensively analyse all of the constructs within the taxonomy | The expected outcome will confirm the key dimensions influencing decision-making and an understanding of user's involvement, rationale and thought processes |
| Phase 3 | Finally, a research model will be developed to determine the causal relationship between the key factors such as user involvement, efficiency, level of persuasion and trust | The research model will demonstrate how the theoretical constructs are positively or negatively impacted by other factors |

This pilot study seeks to address the initial aspect of the second phase of the research plan outlined above. Its purpose is to determine the impact of different decision constructs on decision-making. The focus is on two of the more problematic decision constructs, namely the un-selected and pre-selected opt-out [11]. From the first phase findings, the following key research question emerged: *RQ: How are users impacted by differently designed opt-out decision constructs?*

There are two steps in both parts of the second phase of the research plan:

1. An eye-tracking study where the user's gaze is tracked while completing a simple task using two types of decision constructs, a pre-selected opt-out and an un-selected opt-out. Different presentation options will be used for both pre-selected and un-selected opt-outs (see Table 2). These formats will be based on typical presentation options encountered during the desk analysis described in Sect. 3 and will include pre-selected and un-selected opt-outs. There will be variants of these using different types of framing, both with and without different levels of persuaders (see Table 3). The data gathered includes the user's pattern of eye movement, as well as tracking how long a user focuses on a particular part of the screen. These data allow the researchers to determine how long a user focuses on each of the decision constructs before taking action.

2. Cued retrospective think-aloud sessions where the user talks about the task just completed. The user describes the thought process followed during the task, providing rich, contemporaneous, qualitative data to enhance the quantitative data obtained from eye-tracking. It is important the eye-tracking data is supplemented with additional qualitative data [33], as eye movements simply show the eye movement pattern with no information on why a user is fixating on a particular part of the screen. For example, a long fixation could be due to either interest or difficulty understanding the information.

There are two think-aloud approaches: *concurrent think-aloud* (CTA), where an end user thinks out loud while carrying out tasks on a system, and *retrospective think-aloud* (RTA), where the user provides a description of their thought processes after the tasks have been completed [33]. This verbalization helps the evaluator to understand the user's attitudes towards the system and to identify aspects of the design that are problematic for the user [34]. The sessions are taped and a separate scribe may also take detailed notes of the comments and actions of the user [35]. For this study, CTA was not considered to be an appropriate approach, as it can bias the user's first impression and may influence their visual fixations [36]. RTA also has potential problems, as the user is relying on memory to describe their cognitive processes and may forget information or attempt to justify their actions, leading to erroneous data [37]. However, the use of cued RTA, where the user is shown a playback of their interaction has been found to be more effective at eliciting comments than un-cued RTA [37]. While van den Haak et al. [38] found RTA and CTA identified comparable numbers of usability problems, combining eye-tracking with cued RTA allows the researcher to effectively combine quantitative eye-tracking and qualitative RTA data.

Pernice and Nielsen [30] recommend six users for qualitative eye-tracking (i.e., watching gaze replays). As this pilot is testing the approach before conducting a larger scale study, six users will carry out the tasks while their gaze is tracked using the eye-tracking equipment. They will be shown a replay of their interaction with the gaze pattern superimposed on the screen. While watching the replay, they will describe why they made their decisions and what they were thinking while interacting with the decision constructs. The tasks presented to the users will involve making certain selections using a variety of opt-out decision constructs. These constructs will be both pre-selected and un-selected with the associated information presented in a variety of ways.

Once the pilot tests have been conducted for all participants, the data will be examined in order to plan the analysis for the larger scale study. This will include both quantitative and qualitative analysis. The quantitative analysis will examine the data from the eye-tracking sessions and will determine how the dimensions of option presentation impact on the participants' interaction with the decision constructs. The data examined will include the total interaction time for each webpage; the dwell time (i.e., the sum of all fixation times) for each decision construct; the number of fixations for each interaction; and the mean duration of each fixation. The analysis will consider whether the various dimensions (i.e., default value, framing, persuasion) of the decision construct impact on these times and counts.

The cued RTA sessions will be recorded and notes taken to ensure all data is captured. The qualitative analysis will require an examination of the recorded discussions in order to identify themes and commonalities between the participants', as well as any unique, outlier responses. The data, including responses to prompts as well as any unprompted discourse, will describe participants' thought processes while interacting with the decision constructs. As the cued RTA describes their internal dialogue, this data can help the researchers understand why participants focus on particular parts of the screen. This data will be used to enrich conclusions drawn from the quantitative data and will also allow the researchers determine attitudinal effects of the dimensions of the decision constructs.


## 5   Summary of Research Plan

This paper describes a desk analysis conducted to inform the design for a more comprehensive study gauging the time users spend in examining different types of decision constructs. In addition, the study will explore the rationale and the thought processes in making a decision when users are presented with various types of decision constructs. An in-depth pilot will ensure the study is designed to adequately address the research question. The way in which the decision constructs are presented will be considered, as will issues associated with the cued RTA and eye-tracking itself. The participants will be questioned regarding these issues and others arising during the pilot study.

Once the pilot is complete, a larger study that examines all the previously identified decision constructs will be conducted. It will involve a greater number of participants and will include all decision constructs identified within the taxonomy previously described. This comprehensive study completes phase two of the research plan discussed in Sect. 4.2.

The third phase of the research plan involves composing a research model containing the theoretical constructs along with hypothesized causal associations between the constructs. This study will enhance practitioners and researchers understanding of the impact of decision construct presentation on users' decision-making during the transactional process in B2C interactions.

# References

1. Simon, H.: A Behavioral Model of Rational Choice, in Models of Man, Social and Rational: Mathematical Essays on Rational Human Behavior in a Social Setting. Wiley, New York (1957)
2. Tversky, A., Kahneman, D.: The framing of decisions and the psychology of choices. Science **211**, 453–458 (1981)
3. Samuelson, W., Zeckhauser, R.: Status quo bias in decision making. J. Risk Uncert. **1**(1), 7–59 (1988)
4. Belman, S., Johnson, E., Lohse, G.: To opt-in or opt-out? It depends on the question. Comm. ACM **44**(2), 25–27 (2001)
5. Johnson, E., Goldstein, D.: Do defaults save lives? Science **302**, 1338–1339 (2003)
6. Lai, Y., Hui, K.: Internet opt-in and opt-out: investigating the roles of frames, defaults and privacy concerns. In: Proceedings of SIGMIS-CPR'06, 13–15 Apr, Claremont, California, USA (2006)
7. Torres, A., Barry, C., Hogan, M.: Opaque web practices among low-cost carriers. J. Air Trans. Manag. **15**, 299–307 (2009)
8. European Union: 1008/2008, Regulation of the European Parliament and of the Council on Common Rules for the Operation of Air Services in the Community (Recast) (2008)
9. European Union: 2011/83/EU, Directive on Consumer Rights (2011)
10. Barry, C., Hogan, M., Torres, A.: Perceptions of low cost carriers' compliance with EU legislation on optional extras. In: 20th International Conference on Information Systems Development, 24–26 Aug, Edinburgh, Scotland (2011)
11. Torres, A.M., Barry, C., Hogan, M.: The identification of decision constructs used in online transactional processes. In: 27th Bled eConference, 29 June–3 July, Bled, Slovenia (2014)
12. Hogan, M., Barry, C., Torres, A.: Theorising and testing a taxonomy of decision constructs. J. Cust. Behav. **13**(3), 181–186 (2014)
13. Peter, J.P., Olsen, J.C.: Consumer Behavior: Marketing Strategy Perspectives, Homewood. Irwin, Illinois (1987)
14. Dholakia, U.M.: A motivational process model of product involvement and consumer risk perception. Euro. J. Mark. **35**(11/12), 1340–1360 (2001)
15. Thomsen, C.J., Borgida, E., Lavine, H.: The causes and consequences of personal involvement. In: Petty, R.E., Krosnick, J.A. (eds.) Attitude Strength: Antecedents and Consequences, pp. 191–214. Erlbaum, Mahwah (1995)
16. Trumbo. C.W.: Heuristic-systematic information processing and risk judgment, risk analysis. Int. J. **19**(3), 391–400 (1999)
17. Herrero, A., San Martín, H.: Effects of the risk sources and user involvement on e-Commerce adoption: application to tourist services. J. Risk Res. **15**(7), 841–855 (2012)

18. Moon, S.Y., Philip, G.C., Moon, S.: The effects of involvement on E-Satisfaction models. Serv. Market. Q. **32**(4), 332–342 (2011)
19. Park, D.H., Lee, J., Han, I.: The effect of on-line consumer reviews on consumer purchasing intention: the moderating role of involvement. Int. J. Electron. Comm. **11**(4), 125–148 (2007)
20. MacInnis, D.J., Moorman, C., Jaworski, B.J.: Enhancing and measuring consumers' motivation, opportunity, and ability to process brand information from Ads. J. Market. **55** (4), 32–53 (1991)
21. Johnson, B.T., Eagly, A.H.: The effects of involvement on persuasion: a meta-analysis. Psychol. Bull. **106**(2), 290–314 (1989)
22. Celsi, R.L., Olson, J.C.: The role of involvement in attention and comprehension processes. J. Con. Res. **15**(2), 210–224 (1988)
23. Nielsen, J., Pernice, K.: Eyetracking Web Usability, Fremont. Nielson Norman Group, CA (2009)
24. Djamasbi, S., Siegel, M., Tullis, T., Dai, R.: Efficiency, trust, and visual appeal: usability testing through eye tracking. In: The 43rd Hawaii International Conference on System Sciences (HICSS), pp. 1–10. IEEE (2001)
25. Di Stasi, L., Antoli, A., Gea, M., Canas, J.: A neuroergonomic approach to evaluating mental workload in hypermedia interactions. Int. J. Indus. Erg. **41**, 298–304 (2001)
26. Huang, Y., Kuo, F.: An eye-tracking investigation of internet consumers' decision deliberateness. Internet Res. **21**(5), 541–561 (2011)
27. Sivaji, A., Downe, A., Mazlan, M., Soo, S., Abdullah, A.: Importance of incorporating fundamental usability with social and trust elements for e-Commerce website. In: 2011 International Conference on Business, Engineering and Industrial Applications (ICBEIA), pp. 221–226, IEEE (2011)
28. Djamasbi, S., Siegel, M., Skorinko, J., Tullis, T.: Online viewing and aesthetic preferences of generation Y and the baby boom generation: testing user web site experience through eye tracking. Int. J. Elec. Comm. **15**(4), 121–158 (2011)
29. Goh, K.N., Chen, Y.Y., Lai, F.W., Daud, S.C., Sivaji, A., Soo, S.T.: A comparison of usability testing methods for an E-commerce website: a case study on a Malaysia online gift shop. In: The Tenth International Conference on Information Technology: New Generations (ITNG), pp. 143–150. IEEE (2013)
30. Pernice, K., Nielsen, J.: How to Conduct Eyetracking Studies. http://www.nngroup.com/reports/how-to-conduct-eyetracking-studies/ (2009). Accessed 28 Jan 2015
31. Glöckner, A., Herbold, A.K.: An eye-tracking study on information processing in risky decisions: evidence for compensatory strategies based on automatic processes. J. Behav. Dec. Making **24**, 71–98 (2011)
32. Day, R., Shyi, G., Wang, J.: The effect of flash barriers on multi-attribute decision making: distractor or source of arousal? Psych. Mark. **23**(5), 369–382 (2006)
33. Hyrskykari, A., Ovaska, S., Majaranta, P., Räihä, K.J., Lehtinen, M.: Gaze path stimulation in retrospective think-aloud. J. Eye Mov. Res. **2**(4), 1–18 (2008)
34. Holzinger, A.: Usability engineering methods for software developers. Comm. ACM **48**(1), 71–74 (2014)
35. Monk, A., Wright, P., Haber, J., Davenport, L.: Improving Your Human-Computer Interface A Practical Technique. Prentice Hall, New York (1993)
36. Kim, B., Dong, Y., Kim, S., Lee, K.P.: Development of integrated analysis system and tool of perception, recognition, and behavior for web usability test: with emphasis on eye-tracking, mouse-tracking, and retrospective think aloud. In: Usability and Internationalization. HCI and Culture, pp. 113–121, Springer, Berlin Heidelberg (2007)
37. Ball, L.J., Eger, N., Stevens, R., Dodd, J.: Applying the PEEP method in usability testing. Interfaces **67**, 15–19 (2006)
38. Van den Haak, M.J., de Jong, M.D.T., Schellens, J.: Retrospective vs. concurrent think-aloud protocols: testing the usability of an online library catalogue, Behav. Inf. Tech., **22**(5), pp. 339–351 (2003)

# How Mentorship Improves Reverse Transfer of Tacit Knowledge in Chinese Multinational Companies (MNCs)

Zhenjiao Chen and Dougl Vogel

**Abstract** Knowledge transfer has long been a major focus of research in the literature on MNCs in developed countries. However, reverse knowledge transfer in MNCs in developing countries (e.g., China) has received limited attention. By integrating mentorship, social capital and international adjustment theories, this study develop a theoretical model to demonstrate when and how mentoring improves reverse transfer of tacit knowledge in Chinese MNCs. In particular, we propose that (1) mentoring functions (i.e., vocational support, psychological support and role modelling) should have positive effects on three dimensions of social capital (i.e., ties strength; trust; shared language and vision), which in turn, should improve reverse transfer of tacit knowledge from foreign mentors to Chinese mentees. (2) International adjustment of mentors (i.e., work adjustment, interaction adjustment and general adjustment) is expected to moderate the relationships of mentoring with ties strength, trust, shared language and vision. This is a research-in-progress paper and a survey should be conducted to test the theoretical model. This research should provide theoretical and practical implications.

**Keywords** Reverse transfer of tacit knowledge · Mentoring · Social capital · MNCs · International adjustment

A prior version of this paper has been published in the ISD2015 Proceedings (http://aisel.aisnet.org/isd2014/proceedings2015/).

Z. Chen (✉)
Beijing Institute of Technology, Beijing, China
e-mail: sharon2009@bit.edu.cn

D. Vogel
Harbin Institute of Technology, Harbin, China
e-mail: isdoug@hit.edu.cn

# 1   Introduction

In recent year, statistic report shows that the number of Chinese global M&A ranks second worldwide in 2011, and is expected to exhibit consistent growth in the future [1]. Chinese global M&A aims to improve the "reverse transfer" of tacit knowledge from a foreign subsidiary to the parent company for developing core competitive advantageous and establish Chinese MNCs [1]. Foreign enterprises in developed countries often possess more advanced knowledge than Chinese enterprises [1]. Thus, in MNCs of developing countries (e.g., China), knowledge is often reverse transferred from subsidiaries to a parent company. This differs from traditional knowledge transfer in MNCs of developed countries, in which knowledge is transferred from a parent company to subsidiaries [1].

With the development of Chinese MNCs, reverse knowledge transfer receives more and more attention. Compared with explicit knowledge, tacit knowledge is more pivotal to improve the core competitive advantageous of enterprises, however tacit knowledge is not easily to be transferred [2]. In real business world, reverse transfer of tacit knowledge often fails and results in the failure of many Chinese MNCs and global M&A [1]. Therefore, how to improve reverse transfer of tacit knowledge in Chinese MNCs is pivotal problem need to be solved immediately.

The extant literature mainly focuses on knowledge transfer in MNCs of developed countries, and pays little attention on reverse knowledge transfer in MNCs of developing countries [1]. Moreover, researchers highlight that different types of knowledge have different transfer mechanisms in MNCs; however, rare attention is directed toward the mechanism suitable for tacit knowledge transfer in MNCs [3]. Thus, this study fills this gap to explore how to improve the reverse transfer of tacit knowledge in MNCs of developing countries (e.g., China)?

In knowledge management literature, some scholars focus on the effects of knowledge transfer processes on knowledge transfer effectiveness [4]. Others highlight that knowledge transfer processes is less important than organizational issues, such as incentives, socialization, performance appraisal, communication as well as control and informational mechanisms, in improving knowledge transfer [5–7]. Although the above research found that different types of knowledge had different transfer mechanisms in MNCs [3], they paid little attention on what mechanism was suitable to "tacit knowledge" reverse transfer in MNCs.

Prior research suggests that mentoring, as an organizational issue, could improve tacit knowledge transfer [8]. Tacit knowledge is non-codifiable and is carried by employees from foreign subsidiaries [9]. Thus, a more experienced employee from foreign subsidiaries who carries advanced tacit knowledge can be a mentor and transfer the knowledge to a less experienced employee from the Chinese parent company (the mentee) by direct coaching and interaction behaviors [10, 11]. However, little empirical research has examined the effect of mentoring on reverse knowledge transfer and has explained how mentoring improves the reverse transfer of tacit knowledge in MNCs of developing countries?

Several scholars identified various mediators in a mentorship-outcomes relationship. These mediators include personal learning, role ambiguity and so on [12–14]. In mentoring and coaching, the frequent social interaction between mentors and mentees should elicit the generation of social capital (i.e., potential resources [15] embedded in a mentor-mentee relationship), which benefits knowledge sharing [16]. View in this light, social capital is popular and important in a mentor-mentee relationship; however, no empirical study has examined the mediating role of social capital in the relationship of mentoring with the reverse transfer of tacit knowledge in Chinese MNCs. Thus, the first objective of this study is to adopt social capital theory (SCT) and examine the mediating effect of social capital in the mentoring- tacit knowledge transfer relationship.

Furthermore, in mentorship literature, prior research identified that the mentorship-outcome relationships could be regulated by various moderators, including individual cognition, sex, autonomy, self-efficacy, relational duration and social support [17, 18]. The present research extends the literature by considering the moderating effect of international adjustment on the mentorship-outcomes relationships. In the context of Chinese MNCs, mentoring provided by a foreign mentor might not be clearly understood and absorbed by his/her Chinese mentee because of cultural difference, and therefore deteriorates reverse transfer of tacit knowledge [19]. Thus, the second objective of this study is to explore whether international adjustment, which refers to foreign mentors adapting to Chinese interpersonal interaction style and culture, moderates the relationship between mentoring and reverse transfer of tacit knowledge in Chinese MNCs.

# 2 Literature Review and Research Model

## 2.1 Reverse Transfer of Tacit Knowledge

Knowledge can be categorized as tacit and explicit knowledge. Reverse knowledge transfer refers to a process of the systematic exchange of information and skills from a subsidiary to the parent company in a MNC [1]. In MNCs knowledge transfer literature, one line of research adopts knowledge management theories (e.g., sender-receiver model) to identify factors involved in a knowledge transfer process, such as willingness to transfer, capacity to transfer, capacity to absorb, intent to absorb and knowledge characteristics, as determinants of knowledge transfer [1, 4]. Another line of research adopts organizational behavior theories to identify organizational factors, including incentives, socialization, performance appraisal, communication, control and informational mechanisms, as determinants of knowledge transfer [5–7, 9, 20–23]. These studies have contributed to literature but focused more on general knowledge rather than tacit knowledge, focused more on MNCs of developed countries rather than MNCs of developing counties, and focused more on traditional transfer rather than reverse transfer.

Tacit knowledge is non-codifiable and is difficult to talk and write down. Such knowledge is carried by individuals and can be transferred only through the active involvement of the teachers [21]. Foreign mentors from subsidiaries carrying tacit knowledge may facilitate such reverse transfer through specific coaching behaviors to Chinese mentees in parent companies of Chinese MNCs.

## 2.2  Mentoring and Social Capital

Mentoring is defined as the case in which a more experienced employee (mentor) from subsidiaries who provides a less experienced employee (mentee) from a parent company with technical advice, coaching or information [10].

Prior research found that mentoring had positive effects on various desirable outcomes including learning, organizational knowledge, job satisfaction, organizational commitment, work pressure, performance and career success [10, 13, 24]. Mentoring function includes vocational support, psychosocial support and role modelling [24].

Mentorship is divided into informal mentorship and formal mentorship. The former grows out of an informal relationship and interaction between two organizational members. The latter arises, because an organization requires two organizational members participate into a formal mentorship program. Compared with formal mentorship, mentors in informal mentorship have higher motivation to help their mentees and the mentees are more likely to be open to the assistance of their mentors.

This study focuses on informal mentorship, which develops spontaneously on the basis of perceived competence and interpersonal comfort [24]. A mentor and a mentee in an informal mentorship often have a high quality relationship and have frequent interactions which generate trust and psychosocial functions [24]. These potential resources increase social capital in the mentor-mentee relationship. Thus, this study explores how informal mentoring elicits social capital, which in turn, improves reverse transfer of tacit knowledge.

Based on social capital theory (SCT), social capital refers to the potential resources embedded in and derived from individual relationships [25]. Social capital includes cognitive capital, structural capital and relational capital. Structural capital is manifested as mentor-mentee ties strength (i.e., the degree to which resources, emotional support and time are provided by mentors to mentees) [25]. Relational capital is manifested as trust (i.e., specific beliefs regarding mentors integrity, benevolence and ability) [25]. Cognitive capital is manifested as shared language and shared vision (i.e., shared goals and aspirations) [25]. Prior research focused more on the consequences rather than antecedents of social capital. Only a few of qualitative research explore the antecedents of social capital [26, 27]. For instance, Bolino et al. [26] proposed that organizational citizenship behaviour (OCB) improves social capital. OCB refers to the helping behaviour of employees toward their colleagues [26]. This concept is similar to mentorship, which refers to the helping and coaching behaviour of mentors toward their mentees. Thus, mentoring is expected to improve social capital (ties strength, trust, shared language and vision).

In particular, vocational support indicates that a mentor teaches his/her mentee tacit skills and knowledge through direct coaching or challenging task assignments [11, 24]. During the frequent interaction, the mentor provides lots of resources to the mentee which induces a strong mentor-mentee relation ties. Moreover, the mentor's expertise in vocational support also improves the mentee's trust on the abilities of the mentor. Furthermore, the mentor provides psychosocial support to the mentee through counselling and friendship. The mentee feels free to discuss problems, fears or anxieties with the mentor [11, 24]. Such psychological and emotional support engenders the mentee's trust on his/her mentor benevolence and integrity, as well as leads to a supportive and strong mentor-mentee relationship. In addition, the mentor is also a role model for his/her mentee. Being motivated by the desire to be like and learn from the mentor, the mentee emulate his/her mentor's language, attitudes, values and behaviours [11, 24]. Such practice will induce shared language and shared vision between the mentor and the mentee. Therefore, mentoring is expected to have positive effects on ties strength (structural capital), trust (relational capital) and shared language and vision (cognitive capital).

Meanwhile, SCT claims that individuals can utilize social capital in their social relationships to improve various outcomes [25]. Extant empirical research confirm that structural capital, relational capital and cognitive capital have positive effects on various outcomes, including knowledge transfer, cooperation, organizational knowledge diffusion, informational flow, and so on [26, 28]. Therefore, the above arguments are captured into the following propositions (see Fig. 1):

**Proposition 1a** *Mentoring increases the ties strength (structural capital) of a mentor-mentee relationship, which in turn, improves the reverse transfer of tacit knowledge in Chinese MNCs.*

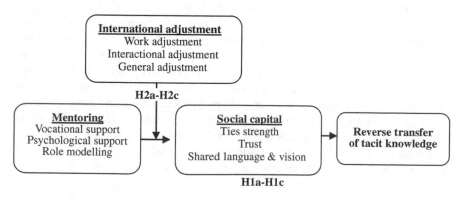

**Fig. 1** Research model

**Proposition 1b** *Mentoring increases trust (relational capital) of a mentor-mentee relationship, which in turn, improves the reverse transfer of tacit knowledge in Chinese MNCs.*

**Proposition 1c** *Mentoring increases shared language and shared vision (cognitive capital) of a mentor-mentee relationship, which in turn, improves the reverse transfer of tacit knowledge in Chinese MNCs.*

## 2.3   Moderating Functions of International Adjustment

Difference in language, thinking, and communication style raises the possibility that the mentoring provided by foreign mentors might not be easily understood by Chinese mentees. This inhibits reverse transfer of tacit knowledge. Thus, this study adopts international adjustment theory (IAT) [29] to identify international adjustment as a new moderator which regulates the effect of mentoring on reverse transfer of tacit knowledge.

In the context of Chinese MNCs, the international adjustment of foreign mentors is defined as the adaptation of foreign mentors to the environment of Chinese MNCs. International adjustment includes three dimensions: task adjustment, which refers to adjustment to job requirements; interactional adjustment, which refers to adjustment to interaction with local Chinese; and general adjustment, which refers to adjustment to Chinese culture [30]. Work adjustment is task-oriented while interactional and general adjustment is relationship-oriented. Interactional adjustment has been found to have positive effects on performance, organizational commitment, job satisfaction, among others [31, 32]. Although the main effect of international adjustment has been well-documented, the moderating function of international adjustment received little attention. This study proposes that international adjustment moderates the mentoring-reverse knowledge transfer relationship. As a foreign mentor with low adjustment always tend to withdraw attention, efforts and resources away from his/her current positions, not even mentioning coaching other colleagues effectively [31]. On the contrary, a well-adjusted foreign mentor often has greater personal resources (time, effort, and emotional investment) and motivation to mentoring his/her mentee efficiently [30].

Firstly, we argued that work adjustment is expected to moderate the effects of mentoring on ties strength and trust. The reason is that only when a foreign mentor has adapted to the new job requirement assigned by a Chinese MNC, can he/she be more likely to spend spare time to provide required coaching and have ability to teach required tacit knowledge to his/her Chinese mentee [30, 31]. The willingness of inputting extra time and resources should improve the mentor-mentee ties strength and make the mentee trust on the mentor's abilities. Secondly, we argue that interactional adjustment moderates the effects of mentoring on ties strength and trust. Given that only a foreign mentor adjusts to Chinese interpersonal interaction style, his/her psychological support could be more appropriate and comfortable for his/her mentees [30, 31]. These conditions could improve the ties strength and trust, respectively. Finally, general adjustment (i.e. mentors' adjustment to Chinese culture) is expected to moderate the effect of mentoring on ties strength, trust, shared vision, and language. The reason is that when a foreign mentor becomes familiar with Chinese culture manifested as language, values, and attitudes, he/she should adapt their attitudes and values according to Chinese culture [30]. The vocational support, psychological support, and role modelling of the mentor could be more effectively absorbed and internalized by the mentee, thus improving ties strength, trust, shared vision and shared language. The above logics can be captured in the following propositions (see Fig. 1):

**Proposition 2a** *Work adjustment moderates the effects of mentoring on ties strength and trust, such that the positive effects of mentoring on ties strength and trust are stronger when work adjustment is high rather than when it is low.*

**Proposition 2b** *Interactional adjustment moderates the effects of mentoring on ties strength and trust, such that the positive effects of mentoring on ties strength and trust are stronger when interactional adjustment is high rather than when it is low.*

**Proposition 2c** *General adjustment moderates the effects of mentoring on ties strength, trust, shared language, and vision, such that the positive effects of mentoring on ties strength, trust, shared language and vision are stronger when general adjustment is high rather than when it is low.*

## 3 Research Site and Data Collection Plan

Data will be collected from 30 Chinese MNCs from diverse industries in diverse districts of China. These 30 MNCs shall represent a convenience sample and will be randomly selected from the list of top 100 Chinese MNCs published by Xinhua News. Human resource (HR) managers of these companies will be contacted to help with survey logistics and to encourage Chinese employees from Chinese parent companies to participate in our survey.

We will provide each Chinese employee with a definition of informal mentoring and then ask a single question about whether he/she has such an informal mentor from the foreign subsidiary. Only the Chinese employees who answer "Yes" will be invited to participate the formal survey to fill in the questionnaire. We will confirm with these mentors. Following many studies of mentoring (for a review, see [10]), we assume that if one half of a mentor-mentee dyad indicates an existing mentoring relation and the other half agrees on it, we will ensure that the mentoring relationship exist. Finally, we plan to invite 1000 Chinese mentees from the 30 parent companies as the respondents of our survey.

We will adopt the temporal separation of measurement approach to reduce common method bias [33] and to provide evidence for the proposed causal directions. Initially, Chinese mentees will complete the items for the control variables and evaluate the mentoring functions of their foreign mentors (independent variable). After approximately one month, they will complete the items to evaluate the international adjustment of their foreign mentors, ties strength, trust, shared language and vision. In the final phase after approximately one month, they will rate the reverse transfer of tacit knowledge. To match the questionnaires completed in different time periods, participants will write their names on the questionnaires. They will be instructed to place the completed questionnaire in sealed envelopes, which will be collected and returned to the researcher directly.

The items for the variables are adopted from the English literature and translated into Chinese by means of a back-translation procedure. Mentoring functions will be measured by 15 items from Lankau and Scandura's research [24] and represent the vocational, psychological, and role modelling dimensions. We will measure ties strength with three items adapted from Dhanaraj and colleagues' research [21]. Trust will be measured using five items from Chiu and colleagues' research [16]. Shared vision and shared language will be measured using three items adapted from Chiu and colleagues' research [16], respectively. Measures for interactional adjustment consist of seven items for general adjustment, four for interaction adjustment, and three for work adjustment adapted from Shaffer et al.'s research [30]. Reverse transfer of tacit knowledge will be measured by three items adapted from Dhanaraj and colleagues' research [21]. A pilot test with a small sample size of 20 Chinese mentees from a MNC will be conducted to test the reliabilities and validities of all measures.

In our study, Chinese indigenous cultural factors such as *guanxi*, *mianzi* and *renqing*, are expected to affect Chinese mentees' behaviours. For instance, for Chinese mentees' with *guanxi* orientation, the psychological support provided by their foreign mentors with high interactional adjustment is more likely to increase the social capital and tacit knowledge transfer. Thus, this research will identified mentees' *guanxi* orientation, *mianzi* orientation and *renqing* orientation as control variables.

Data will be analysed by SPSS and LISREL 8.70. In particular, descriptive analysis of the sample, reliability and validity of measure will be tested by SPSS. The measurement model will be tested by LISREL. Propositions of mediating and moderating effects will be tested by Sobel test and moderation analysis of SPSS, respectively.

# 4  Discussion

This research-in-progress study presents a theoretical model to investigate how mentoring affects the reverse transfer of tacit knowledge in Chinese MNCs. A preliminary analysis of the literature review suggests that most previous research has focused on knowledge transfer in MNCs of developed countries, with less attention directed toward reverse tacit knowledge transfer in MNCs of developing countries. Considering the tacitness of knowledge, we propose that mentoring could be an effective mechanism for the reverse transfer of tacit knowledge from subsidiaries to parent companies in Chinese MNCs. Moreover, considering cultural difference, we propose that the international adjustment of mentors could be a moderator in the mentoring-reverse tacit knowledge transfer relationship. By integrating SCT and IAT, our research model presents when and how mentoring affects reverse tacit knowledge transfer in Chinese MNCs, that is, mentoring improves reverse tacit knowledge transfer through eliciting three dimensions of social capital. Moreover, the mediating processes are expected to be regulated by international adjustment. We believe that this novel perspective offers theoretical contribution to mentoring and knowledge management literature. What's more, our research findings should enlighten knowledge management practitioners in Chinese MNCs.

**Acknowledgements** This study is sponsored by the National Natural Science Foundation of China (71471017); Beijing Higher Education Young Elite Teacher Project (Principal Investigator: Z.J. Chen, No. YETP1164, 3210036521404), Beijing Excellent Talents Fund (Principal Investigator: Z.J. Chen, No. 2013D009011000006, 3210036521407); Basic Research Fund of Beijing Institute of Technology (Principal Investigator: Z.J. Chen, No. 20132142005, 3210012211405). 2012 Science and Technology Project Funds for Oversea Scholars (Principal Investigator: Z.J. Chen, No. 3210036821201).

# References

1. Liu, M.X.: Reverse Knowledge Transfer in Chinese MNCs. Chinese Social Science Press, Beijing (2012)
2. Lazarova, M., Tarique, I.: Knowledge transfer upon repatriation. J. World Bus. **40**, 361–373 (2005)
3. Foss, N.J., Pedersen, T.: Transferring knowledge in MNCs: the role of sources of subsidiary knowledge and organizational context. J. Int. Manag. **8**, 49–67 (2002)
4. Najafi-Tavani, Z., Giroud, A., Sinkovics, R.R.: Mediating effects in reverse knowledge transfer process: the case of knowledge-intensive services in the U.K. Manag. Int. Rev. **52**, 461–488 (2012)
5. Gupta, A.K., Govindarajan, V.: Knowledge flows within multinational corporations. Strateg. Manag. J. **21**, 473–496 (2000)
6. Persson, M.: The impact of operational structure, lateral integrative mechanisms and control mechanisms on intra-MNE knowledge transfer. Int. Bus. Rev. **15**, 547–569 (2006)
7. Schotter, A., Bontis, N.: Intra-organizational knowledge exchange: an examination of reverse capability transfer in multinational corporations. J. Intellect. Capital **10**, 149–164 (2009)
8. Swap, W., Leonard, D., Shields, M., Abrams, L.: Using mentoring and storytelling to transfer knowledge in the workplace. J. Manag. Inf. Syst. **18**, 95–114 (2001)
9. Fang, Y., Jiang, F., Makino, S., Beamish, P.W.: Multinational firm knowledge, use of expatriates, and foreign subsidiary performance. J. Manage. Stud. **47**, 27–54 (2010)
10. Carraher, S., Sullivan, S., Crocitto, M.: Mentoring across global boundaries: an empirical examination of home- and host-country mentors on expatriate career outcomes. J. Int. Bus. Stud. **39**, 310–326 (2008)
11. Kram, K.E.: Mentoring at Work: Developmental Relationships in Organizational Life. Scott, Foresman, Glenview, IL (1985)

12. Blickle, G., Witzki, A.H., Schneider, P.B.: Mentoring support and power: a three year predictive field study on protégé networking and career success. J. Vocat. Behav. **74**, 181–189 (2009)
13. Haggard, D., Dougherty, T., Turban, D., Wilbanks, J.: Who is a mentor? A review of evolving definitions and implications for research. J. Manag. **37**, 280–306 (2011)
14. Payne, S.C., Huffman, A.H.: A longitudinal examination of the influence of mentoring on organizational commitment and turnover. Acad. Manag. J. **48**, 158–168 (2005)
15. Coleman, J.S.: Social capital in the creation of human capital. Am. J. Sociol. **94**, 95–120 (1988)
16. Chiu, C.M., Hsu, M.H., Wang, T.G.: Understanding knowledge sharing in virtual communities: an integration of social capital and social cognitive theories. Decis. Support Syst. **42**, 1872–1888 (2006)
17. Larose, S., Tarabulsy, G., Cyrenne, D.: Perceived autonomy and relatedness as moderating the impact of teacher-student mentoring relationships on student academic adjustment. J. Primary Prevent. **26**, 1–22 (2005)
18. Norziani, N., Ahmad, Z.: Learning from informal mentor and self-efficacy: the moderating role of social support. Int. J. Knowl. Cult. Change Manage. **5**, 161–168 (2010)
19. Yu, P.: Knowledge transfer within multinational companies. Doctoral thesis, Shang Dong University (2006)
20. Bjorkman, I., Barner-Rasmussen, W., Li, L.: Managing knowledge transfer in MNCs: the impact of headquarters control mechanisms. J. Int. Bus. Stud. **35**, 443–455 (2004)
21. Dhanaraj, C., Lyles, M.A., Steensma, H.K., Tihanyi, L.: Managing tacit and explicit knowledge transfer in IJVs: the role of relational embeddedness and the impact on performance. J. Int. Bus. Stud. **35**, 428–442 (2004)
22. Piscitello, L., Rabbiosi, L.: How does knowledge transfer from foreign subsidiaries affect parent companies' innovative capacity. Druid Working Paper. **10**, 06–22 (2006)
23. Rabbiosi, L.: The evolution of reverse knowledge transfer within multinational corporations. Working Paper, Politecnico di Milano, Milan (2005)
24. Lankau, M.J., Scandura, T.A.: An investigation of personal learning in mentoring relationships: content, antecedents, and consequences. Acad. Manag. J. **45**, 779–790 (2002)
25. Nahapiet, J., Ghoshal, S.: Social capital, intellectual capital and the organizational advantage. Acad. Manag. Rev. **23**, 242–266 (1998)
26. Bolino, M.C., Turnley, W.H., Bloodgood, J.M.: Citizenship behavior and the creation of social capital in organizations. Acad. Manag. Rev. **27**, 505–522 (2002)
27. Fang, R., Duffy, M.K., Shaw, J.D.: The organizational socialization process: review and development of a social capital model. J. Manag. **37**, 127–152 (2011)
28. Maurer, I., Bartsch, V., Ebers, M.: The value of intra-organizational social capital: how it fosters knowledge transfer, innovation performance, and growth. Organ. Stud. **32**, 157–185 (2011)
29. Black, J.S., Mendenhall, M., Oddou, G.: Toward a comprehensive model of international adjustment: an integration of multiple theoretical perspectives. Acad. Manag. Rev. **16**, 291–317 (1991)
30. Shaffer, M.A., Harrison, D.A., Gilley, K.M.: Dimensions, determinants, and differences in the expatriate adjustment process. J. Int. Bus. Stud. **30**, 557–581 (1999)
31. Bhaskar-Shrinivas, P., Harrison, D.A., Shaffer, M.A., Luk, D.M.: Input-based and time-based models of international adjustment: meta-analytic evidence and theoretical extensions. Acad. Manag. J. **48**, 257–281 (2005)
32. Hechanova, R., Beehr, T.A., Christiansen, N.D.: Antecedents and consequences of employees' adjustment to overseas assignment: a meta-analytic review. Appl. Psychol. **52**, 213–236 (2003)
33. Podsakoff, P.M., MacKenzie, S.B., Lee, J., Podsakoff, N.P.: Common method biases in behavioral research: a critical review of the literature and recommended remedies. J. Appl. Psychol. **88**, 879–903 (2003)

# Optimal Requirements—Dependent Model-Driven Agent Development

**Joshua Z. Goncalves and Aneesh Krishna**

**Abstract** The Belief-Desire-Intention (BDI) agent architecture is a favored agent development architecture known for its distinct abstraction between components and flexibility in determining its actions. This determination is handled through a plan selection function which determines the most appropriate plan or action. Recent years have seen various forms of extensions to this architecture, including a model-driven creation approach based around the Extended Non-functional requirements framework (ENFR). Non-functional requirements illustrate parts of a system which must be satisfied to an appropriate extent. The model-driven approach within this paper uses components from this framework to formulate plans governed by their contribution to these requirements. This is done in an optimized manner to ensure the selected plan is optimal with regards to the systems attainment. This paper presents our optimized model-driven agent development approach, demonstrating its conversion from the initial ENFR model into a completely optimized agent. The approach is verified through empirical analysis.

## 1 Introduction

Autonomous agents are steadily becoming a viable solution for various applications in the industry due to their high level of adaptability and flexibility. This makes them a more appropriate alternative to traditional software implementations depending on the context [1]. Creating these agents however has long been a difficult feat in modern software engineering, with their implementation and

A prior version of this paper has been published in the ISD2015 Proceedings (http://aisel.aisnet.org/isd2014/proceedings2015/).

J.Z. Goncalves (✉) · A. Krishna
Department of Computing, Curtin University, Bentley, WA 6102, Australia
e-mail: joshua.goncalves@student.curtin.edu.au

A. Krishna
e-mail: A.Krishna@curtin.edu.au

© Springer International Publishing Switzerland 2016
D. Vogel et al. (eds.), *Transforming Healthcare Through Information Systems*,
Lecture Notes in Information Systems and Organisation 17,
DOI 10.1007/978-3-319-30133-4_10

135

approach being application-specific. This is mainly due to the expertise required in both their actual implementation and the methodology/design approach required to create them successfully.

With the rise in popularity of the Belief-Desire-Intention (BDI) architecture [2], this agent creation process has become conceptually easier. Currently, there exists a multitude of techniques [3, 4] which rely and build upon it as well as accompanying platforms [5, 6] which implement it. Regardless of this however, the entry-level knowledge requirement is still high, with many developers understandably choosing to stick with a comfortable alternative as opposed to the economic risk. In light of this, model-driven agent development (MDD) [7] frameworks (such as the one in this paper) are being explored to reduce the agent-oriented aspects into the background. This means that the developer only needs to focus on the traditional programming aspects. This allows agent-oriented technology to reach a larger audience due to this reduced complexity, being applicable to a wider range of fields which would not have previously considered it.

Our approach is based on the Extended Non-Functional Requirements (ENFR) framework [8, 9] which uses the original NFR-framework but replaces the qualitative reasoning to instigate a quantitative approach, allowing determinism. Our approach uses the preferences given to operationalizations within the ENFR model as well as the progressive values of its children to determine which operationalization is the most appropriate. This means that the selected operationalization is optimal both by itself and the potential path it can take through its children. Using this approach, and based on any combination of operationalizations available at a particular moment, the optimal path with respect to both time and space complexity will be followed. This means that, despite the approach's model foundations, agents created from it will perform optimally, allowing newer audiences to reap the benefits usually aligned only with traditionally developed agents.

In the next section (Sect. 2), we provide background knowledge on both the BDI agent architecture and the Extended NFR framework as well as other work related to this research. In Sect. 3 we provide an explanation of the development and methodology surrounding our optimized model-driven agent creation approach. In Sect. 4 we present our optimization model mathematically, including how it functions and proof of its optimality. In Sect. 5 we evaluate our optimized approach empirically against static, random, and preferential-based approaches and finally, in Sect. 6, we conclude the paper.

## 2    Background

### 2.1    Belief-Desire-Intention Agent Framework

The BDI Agent framework specifies a certain structure which enables agent creation in a conceptually adept, flexible, and powerful manner. A practical agent implemented using this framework is basically a dynamic planning system that determines which plans to execute in order to achieve its goals [2]. BDI agents are conceptually split into three different parts, as denoted by their acronym. Beliefs represent information from the agent itself, its environment, and other agents that it communicates with. Internally, these beliefs are represented as variables with their value denoting the state of the belief. Desires are objectives which the agent strives to achieve. These are represented as goals which can be triggered by both the agent itself and by perceptions received from the agents own environment. Intentions represent a series of pre-defined actions which the agent has decided to take in order to make a chosen desire or series of desires true. These are represented as plans which the agent is capable of performing. In order to satisfy some desires, multiple plans following a sequence are necessary.

We now describe a typical execution cycle from a BDI agent following a default implementation. Initially, the BDI agent will receive a perception (created either internally or from its environment) which will trigger a range of possible plans. The triggered plans will then have their various execution conditions checked to create a further subset of applicable plans. From this subset, a plan is chosen and executed. This plan selection strategy is known as the plan selection function which determines the plan that is most appropriate from the range of available plans given the agent's context and percept sequence to date.

## 2.2  Extended NFR Framework

The extended NFR-framework revolves around two main entities, which are softgoals and operationalizations. Softgoals represent non-functional requirements, which are requirements that cannot be determinatively satisfied such as performance. Each softgoal has a numerical weighting which determines its importance. Operationalizations are ways of satisfying these softgoals. For example, by achieving operationalizations with regards to the performance softgoal, it can be seen that the system will be fast. Both of these components can be decomposed into child variations.

Each apex operationalization makes a contribution to a leaf softgoal which represents the operationalization's impact on that softgoal. These contributions are each given a value to denote their magnitude. This value, multiplied by the softgoal's weighting, creates a summation which becomes the respective operationalization's score. The operationalizations with positive scores are then selected to be implemented into the system, since this positivity means that they are beneficial. From the set of selected operationalizations, the attainment of the overall system can then be calculated. This attainment score represents the degree at which all softgoals within the system have been satisfied. Due to content constraints, this framework will not be detailed further, please refer to its respective papers [8, 10] for more information if required.

## 2.3  Related Work

Softgoal-based plan selection is a softgoal-based approach to agent plan selection [11] implemented through BDI4JADE [5]. Softgoal-based plan selection uses a series of softgoals and plans, with contributions shared between them. The agent is evolved from a declared meta-model, utilizing these components through a model-driven approach. There are two key differences between this and our approach. The first difference is that they do not consider their child plans when selecting a plan, basing their selection on only what the agent can currently access. This leads to plan selection that is suboptimal, resulting in their approach selecting plans which may not necessarily be the best choice. The second key difference is the intended environment of the agent. Our approach was built around the idea of performing in a dynamic environment where perceptions may change the agent's belief base. Their approach does not consider such an environment, assuming that their environment is static so that their belief state will not change throughout the agent's lifetime. Given this static set of base knowledge, their agent can be considered an abstraction of a reflex agent. These agents cannot operate in an environment unless it is static and discrete. This limits their agents drastically in comparison to ours, which is a derivative of a utility agent, such that it can cope within dynamic environments by modifying its belief state to suit any changes [12].

Our approach to designing agents is a Process-oriented one, not unlike agent methodologies such as Prometheus [13]. Prometheus is a standard planning-to-implementation approach to designing agents. Prometheus ventures into detail about creating various entities in a structured approach. This means that the objects are created in earlier stages and are progressively abstracted less and less until they can be implemented. Our approach is much more light-weight in comparison, along with being more accessible and modifiable without having to adhere to harsh design constraints. This however, means that our approach is also very static in the agents that it can create. Although they can fulfil many uses, they are constrained due to their model-based foundations. Using Prometheus, one can create a wider range of agents, albeit with much more overhead compared to our approach, and requiring expert knowledge.

## 3  Optimized Model-Driven Agent Development

### 3.1  ENFR-to-Agent Mapping

From the original ENFR diagram, various components of it can be directly mapped to our agent. This starts with the belief state of the agent. The agent's belief state consists of an abstracted version of the ENFR model, containing all of the components and relationships within it. This means that each operationalization and

**Table 1** Mapping rules

| Mapping rule | Transformation |
|---|---|
| Agent | Load ENFR graph structure |
| | Initialize operationalization scores |
| | Perform preliminary propagation |
| Plan | Operation ← specific operationalization |
| | Precondition ← comparison value |
| Softgoal | Initialize softgoal object and set its weighting and identifier |
| Operationalization | Initialize operationalization object |
| | Set probability and identifier in new object |
| | Initialize operationalization parent, children and softgoal links |

softgoal gets their own objects containing their relationships and values. These objects are arranged in a tree-structure within the system, providing quick traversal and access to each of them.

The mapping of plans within the agent starts with System plans, which are trigger points in the agent based on a series of softgoals. Based on a series of perceptions, a system plan will be executed. This plan will then create goals which will trigger the subsequent operation plans. Each operationalization within the agent gets their own operation plan, whose computation relates to the operationalization's purpose. Within these plans exists the relevant operationalization object as well as the plans preference, which is its operationalization's score multiplied by its probability of success. By including the operationalization object, any changes to the belief state that relates to this operationalization can be automatically incorporated by the plan. Softgoals within the agent are represented only by their object and are not mapped to an explicit BDI agent component. An abstracted version of this mapping can be seen in Table 1.

Using the above mapping, we now detail how a typical execution cycle occurs. The agent initially detects a series of perceptions from its environment. Using these perceptions, it triggers a system plan. The system plan will then trigger a goal based on its represented softgoals. The operation plan(s) contributing to these softgoals are then triggered by this goal, with the plan selection function executing the most beneficial one amongst them. Once this plan has finished its computation, it will reference the agent to trigger its children, with respect to the relationship that it has with them.

## 3.2 Optimization Preparation

When deciding between a series of operation plans, the agent ideally wants to select the plan which will achieve the highest level of attainment for the overall system. This is in relation not just to the plan itself, but also to any children which it may have and the optimal selection amongst them. This is because the parent operation plan is dependent on the completion of its children. Therefore, if the children's completion probability is low, or their operationalization has negative contributions, then the overall benefit achieved by their parent will be effected. In order to handle this, our optimization procedure adds two additional values to each operation plan. The first is the Preview value which is a percentage that represents the degree of change between the operation plans preference and the average preferences of its children. The second value is the Preview Depth which represents the number of child operation plans participating in the optimal path, including itself. By multiplying the preview value against the plans preference, we reach the Comparison Value. This value represents the degree of benefit from the most optimal path taken from the current point.

Creating the preview value is done through two forms of propagation, depending on the situation. The first is the preliminary propagation which occurs once the agent has been created. For each apex operation plan, its preview value is created by propagating downwards to its leaf-child plans. Once these children have been reached, their preview value and preview depth are calculated, which, considering that they have no children, will both be one. It then moves upwards to their parents and calculates their preview value. This is done by, for each of the parent's children depending on their relationship, calculating their original average by multiplying their preview value by their own preference value. A summation for all of these child averages is then created, with the parent's preference value being added to it as well. A summation for the children's preview depths is created alongside this, being incremented to include the parent. The summation of the child preview values is then divided by the summation of the preview depths and then further divided by the parent's preference to create its preview value. This continues for every parent until the original apex operation plans have been reached. The second form of propagation is from an operation plan upwards through its parents. This is to increase efficiency, since if this operation plan is modified, then the only preview values effected are its own and its parents. This process is the same as the initial propagation method.

Within both propagations, the relationship shared between the parent and child must be observed, which is either inclusive or exclusive. Within an inclusive relationship, the preview values of all children must be taken into account. This is because, when initializing the parents preview value, each child must be executed in order to complete it. For exclusive relationships, only the child with the largest comparison value needs to be considered, because the most optimal path from the parent occurs through this child. This process can be seen in Algorithm 1.

```
Algorithm 1: PreviewPropagation(OperationPlan operation)
Input: operation: Operation plan whose preview value
needs to be determined/updated
preview = 0, tempValue = 0, operation.previewDepth = 1;
  for each child in operation.children do
    if child.comparisonValue > tempValue AND
       relationship = OR then
       operation.previewDepth = child.previewDepth + 1
       preview = child.comparisonValue  child.previewDepth
       tempValue = child.comparisonValue
    else
       tempValue = child.comparisonValue
         child.previewDepth
       preview += tempValue
       operation.previewDepth += child.previewDepth
    end if
  end for
preview = (preview + operation.preference)/
  operation.previewDepth
operation.previewValue = preview / operation.preference
```

## 3.3  Operation Plan Selection Function

When creating our plan selection function, establishing a simple and efficient method of operation plan comparison was the main focus. However, we also had to adhere to the dynamic environment that our agents were developed to thrive in. This means that, as well as handling the comparison between operation plans, we also needed to refresh their values in the scenario that a change occurred. We achieved this by separating our function into two main areas. The first handles the re-initialization of an operation plan. This consists of creating a summation of the operationalization's contributions (multiplied by the recipient softgoal's weighting) as well as the scores of its parent operationalizations. This score is then multiplied by the operation plans success probability to result in its preference. If any changes occurred prior to the execution of this operation plan, then they will be captured within this new value. The second area is the actual comparison of the value itself. This process consists of initially calculating the operation plans comparison value, which takes both the probability and quality of the operation plans children into account. This value is then compared with the same computation from other operation plans and the one with the highest value is selected. This process can be seen further within Algorithm 2.

```
Algorithm 2: OptimizedPlanSelection(OperationPlanSet
operationSet)
Input: operationSet: set of considered operation plans
preference = 0, tempValue = 0, tempPlan = NULL;
for each operation ∈ operationSet do
      for each c ∈ operation.contributions do
        preference = preference + (c.softgoalWeight
          c.value)
      end for
      for each op ∈ operation.parents do
        preference = preference + op.score
      end for
      operation.preference = preference
        operation.probability
      preference = 0
end for
for each operation ∈ operationSet do
  if (operation.preference  operation.previewValue) >
    tempValue then
    tempValue = operation.preference
      operation.previewValue
    tempPlan = operation
  end if
end for
tempPlan.execute()
```

## 4  Optimization Model

### 4.1  Model Calculations

For a given ENFR network N, the associated variables are calculated as follows:

*Base Preference*: The preference of an operation plan without the preview value being taken into consideration. The calculation is based on the operationalization's contributions to softgoals (respective to their weighting) as well as any parent operationalizations it may have. The base preference is calculated below with Eq. 1a calculating the original preference value and Eq. 1b applying the probability to it.

$$basePref = \sum_{SG_i \in SG} (contr_i \cdot W_i) + \sum_{pOP_j \in OP} basePref_j \qquad (1a)$$

$$basePref = basePref \cdot probability, \quad 0 \leq probability \geq 1 \quad (1b)$$

where SG is a set of leaf-softgoals, W is the softgoal's weighting and pOP is a set of parent operationalizations.

*Preview Value*: The preview value is calculated using two variations to account for inclusive and exclusive relationships. The propagation elements of these variations are shown below with a generalized preview calculation shown after in Eq. 4a, b.

*Inclusive*: Eq. 2a, b calculates the inclusive propagation elements of the preview value. Equation 2a cycles through the operation plan's children to calculate a cumulative average amongst them. Equation 2b does the same but in relation to the children's depth, determining how many child plans exist throughout the relationship.

$$preview = \sum_{cOP_i \epsilon OP_j} (comparisonV_i \cdot previewDepth_i) \quad (2a)$$

$$previewDepth = \left( \sum_{cOP_i \in OP} previewDepth_i \right) + 1 \quad (2b)$$

where cOP is a set of child operation plans.

*Exclusive*: Eq. 3a, b calculates the exclusive propagation elements of the preview value. Equation 3a cycles through the operation plan's children to determine the maximum comparison value amongst them. Equation 3b calculates the preview depth value based on the operation plan selected previously.

$$preview = \max(comparisonV_i \cdot previewDepth_i), \quad \forall OP_i \in cOP \quad (3a)$$

$$previewDepth = previewDepth_i + 1 \quad (3b)$$

*Generalized Preview*: Eq. 4a, b calculates the final preview value and preview depth value for an operation plan j based on the above propagation elements. Equation 4a calculates the preview value for the operation plan. Equation 4b calculates the preview depth for the operation plan.

$$preview_j = \left( \frac{preview + basePref_j}{previewDepth_j} \right) / basePref_j \quad (4a)$$

$$previewDepth_j = previewDepth \quad (4b)$$

*Comparison Value*: The Comparison value is calculated based on the preview value and the base preference of the operation plan, as seen in Eq. 5.

$$comparisonV = basePref \cdot preview \tag{5}$$

*Ideal Attainment*: This optimization model is based on the idea of maximizing the ENFR networks overall attainment. The ideal attainment score, calculated in Eq. 6, represents a perfect system where all softgoals can be completely satisfied. Since not all softgoals may be applicable based on the received perceptions, this only concerns the ones which are contained within the current selection. This is because any subset of operation plans can be considered for execution at any one moment.

$$A_{ideal} = \sum_i LSGw_{(i)}, \quad \forall LSG_i \in Selection \tag{6}$$

*Actual Attainment:* The actual attainment score represents a system where not all softgoals can be completely satisfied. Given perfect satisfiability is unachievable, the highest possible satisfiability must be used instead, which is achieved through operation plan j, as seen in Eq. 7.

$$ComparisonV_i = Max(Min(ComparisonV_j, 1), -1), \quad \forall LSG_i \in Selection \tag{7}$$

$$A_{actual} = \sum_i \left( LSGw_{(i)} \cdot \left( contri_{(ji)} \cdot comparisonV_j \right) \right)$$

where contr(ji) is a contribution from an operation plan's represented operationalization j to a softgoal i and Selection is the series of softgoals relevant to the current environment of the agent. In order to achieve the full contribution, *comparisonV_j* must be equal or larger than one. Any value less and the full contribution will not be achieved.

## 4.2   Mathematical Proof

Using the ideal and actual attainment scores, the current optimization model can be expanded into its singular elements, which are the operation plan's children, and proven. This proof can be seen detailed below.

$$A_{actual} = \sum_i \left( LSGw_{(i)} \cdot \left( contr_{ji} \cdot comparisonV_j \right) \right)$$

$$A_{actual}/A_{ideal} = \sum_i \left( \frac{LSGw_{(i)} \cdot \left( contr_{ji} \cdot comparisonV_j \right)}{LSGw_{(i)}} \right)$$

$$= \sum_i \left( contr_{ji} \cdot comparisonV_j \right), where\ contr_{ji} = constant\ C$$

$$= \sum_i \left( comparisonV_j \right)$$

$$comparisonV = basePref \cdot preview = \frac{basePref \cdot preview}{basePref}$$

$$comparisonV = preview$$

$$preview = \frac{preview + basePref}{previewDepth} = \frac{comparisonV + basePref}{previewDepth}$$

$$= \frac{\left( comparisonV \cdot previewDepth \right) + basePref}{previewDepth}$$

$$= \sum_{i=n}^{0} \frac{comparisonV_i + basePref_i}{previewDepth_i} = basePref, \quad previewDepth = 1$$

$$comparisonV = basePref \cdot \frac{\sum_{i=n}^{0} basePref_n/previewDepth_n}{basePref}$$

$$= \sum_{i=n}^{0} basePref_n/previewDepth_n$$

$$= Avg(basePref), \quad \forall cOP \in sOP\ Selection$$

This process results in the actual attainment being reduced to the average of the base preferences from all the operation plans along a path starting from the initial operation plans such that:

$$max(A_{actual}) \propto max(Avg(basePref)), \quad \forall cOP \in pOP \in Selection$$

This proves that, in order to achieve the maximum attainment for the system, the operation plan and its children which have the highest base preferences must be chosen. By basing the optimization model around the averages of subsequent operation plan children, this is easily achievable.

# 5  Evaluation

Now that we have detailed our optimization model and how the agent can use it to achieve optimality, we will evaluate our optimization approach empirically. Our approach, based on the operation plan's preference relative to its children, should always choose the optimal path of plans regardless of the underlying ENFR network's configuration. To test this declaration, we perform static, random, preferential and our optimized plan selection approach on a set example. The settings of this experiment are shown in Sect. 5.1 with the results and prompt discussion shown in Sects. 5.2 and 5.3 respectively.

## 5.1  Experiment Settings

Our experiment consists of a simulation that compares the satisfaction achieved in the system when a specific plan is selected using each of the methods, beginning with a fresh ENFR network configuration. This configuration will then be randomly changed throughout the agent's execution in order to emulate a dynamic environment. The evaluation will consist of four distinct approaches. The first is a static approach which comes in two variations, one which selects the first operation plan and another which selects the last. The second approach is completely random, selecting a random operation plan from the available selection, regardless of scoring. The third approach is the preferential approach which selects an operation plan based on its preference alone, independent to its children. The final approach is our optimized approach, which selects an operation plan based on its preference and the preferences of its children.

The simulation scenario is very similar to the banking system seen within the ENFR literature [8, 10], except it has been extended to allow for a more stressful evaluation. It was chosen because of its appropriate understandability, allowing for easy reproduction of the evaluation and its results. Throughout this simulation, the agent must constantly make decisions upon which operation plans it should execute to ensure the success of the system in relation to a series of softgoals. These softgoals are as follows:

- Space
- Response Time
- Data Security
- Accuracy
- Confidentiality
- Memory Retainment
- Availability
- User-Friendly

Using the model defined above, each operation plan has different contributions (if any) to a subsection of these softgoals. Due to the sheer size of the model, these contributions will not be explicitly stated. Our experiment consists of the following steps after the ENFR network generation:

1. Select an appropriate operation plan using all prior mentioned approaches.
2. Evaluate the attainment of this selection using the optimization approach detailed in Sect. 4.1, which measures optimality based on the comparison value of the selected operation plan.
3. Modify the ENFR network configuration by replacing a softgoal's weighting, operationalization's contribution to a softgoal, or an operation plan's probability with a randomly generated value.

Evaluation of each approach will be based on the same triggered goals and dynamic changes in order to ensure a fair experiment.

## 5.2 Results and Analysis

In our experiment, we ran 1000 iterations of the steps described above. This number was chosen arbitrarily to provide an indicative, traceable measure of the performance of our approach, with the results being entirely independent to it. Each iteration took a fixed 0.1 s to run due to threading considerations, with the performance being well under this with the limitations removed.

For each iteration, we noted the comparison value achieved by the selected operation plan, since this value denotes the operation plan's overall benefit to the system. This information was summarized for each approach and presented in a more distinguishable form. This includes the maximum, minimum, mean, median, standard deviation and variation scores. The raw scores are shown in Table 2, with a supporting visual box-plot in Fig. 1.

As evident, on average, our optimized approach had the highest attainment rate, while the remaining approaches had less than satisfactory results. This means that, even with constant, dynamic changes being applied to the agent, our approach was still able to reliably select the optimal plan to achieve the maximum attainment. We

**Table 2** Evaluation results (n = 1000)

| Approach | Min | Max | Mean | Median | SD | V |
|----------|-----|-----|------|--------|-----|---|
| Optimized | −0.04762 | 2.298 | 0.26157 | 0.21108 | 0.23284 | 0.05421 |
| Preferential | −0.04762 | 2.298 | 0.25664 | 0.20717 | 0.23234 | 0.05398 |
| Static left | −0.07004 | 1.59383 | 0.19182 | 0.14155 | 0.18254 | 0.03332 |
| Static right | −0.04762 | 1.59383 | 0.18588 | 0.13250 | 0.17711 | 0.03137 |
| Random | −0.07004 | 1.65124 | 0.18657 | 0.12743 | 0.19183 | 0.03680 |

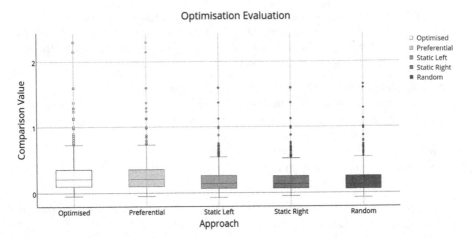

**Fig. 1** Evaluation box-plot (n = 1000)

will now examine the results achieved by exploring each notable measure sequentially.

The minimum and maximum values across the experiment were 0.07004 and 2.298 respectively. Our optimized approach achieved the maximum value and also achieved the highest minimum value of 0.04762. This means that, in both the best-case and worst-case scenarios, our optimized approach performed optimally, especially in comparison to the other approaches.

The highest mean value achieved across the experiment was 0.26157, which was achieved uniquely by our optimized approach and was 29 % higher than the smallest average. This data indicates that, during the experiment, the operation plans chosen by our optimized approach achieved higher attainment in comparison to all other approaches. This includes the preferential approach, which achieved a mean value of 0.25664. This demonstrates that our optimized approach surpasses a similar approach which bases itself only on the current operation plans, irrespective of their children. Although this increase is only 2 %, given larger models and a higher branching factor, this gap could increase exponentially.

The smallest standard deviation achieved across the experiment was 0.17711 from a static approach. Our optimized approach in comparison achieved a standard deviation of 0.23284, which is 24 % higher. This entails that our approach is not as consistent with its values in comparison to the other approaches. And whilst this is empirically correct, within our agent's dynamic environment, this inconsistency is something that is favored. It means that our agent selected values between cycles that greatly differed from each other. Since each cycle has a different set of available operation plans to choose from, and a new modification to the underlying ENFR network, this inconsistency is a trait of optimality. To achieve consistency would be to select the worst value in every scenario since value degradation is more consistent that improvement. Therefore, having the largest standard deviation from the experiment is supportive of the optimality demonstrated by our optimized approach.

## 5.3  Discussion

As discussed above, in all iterations, our optimized approach selected the optimal path. Compared to the other approaches, this means that our approach achieved the highest level of attainment consistently, given its dynamic context.

As well as optimality, our experiment also gave us a platform to compare the technical performance of the approaches. The optimized and preferential approaches both had a time complexity of $O(s)$, due to the initial plan comparisons, where $s$ refers to the number of plans under consideration. This is slightly larger than the time complexity of the remaining approaches, which have a minimum time complexity of $O(1)$. Given the way our agent operates however, this difference is negligent. This is because this difference is dependent entirely on the underlying ENFR model where the number of plans originates from. Given that only a subset of these plans can be selected initially (contributing plans) and a further subset of these plans exist for selection (applicable plans), even large ENFR models will have little effect in terms of time complexity. This is evident through the results, which had indistinguishable timing for each approach, aligning with the processing constraints commonly required by agent technology.

Our experiment also allowed us to identify a limitation of our approach which is with regards to the way the preview values are expressed, which is as a percentage. By expressing the preview in this manner, some ENFR model changes do not require propagation to maintain preview accuracy. This is because the ratio between the new preference and its children remains static. However, when the represented operationalizations of children of an operation plan contribute to a softgoal, this addition can cause the ratio to become inaccurate. Although this is rectified naturally through agent computation, the cycles required to do so may possibly inhibit optimality by a minuscule amount for a brief duration. Rectifying this would cause the agent to perform propagation in scenarios where it is not necessarily required. Due to the additional computation this would require, it is currently not considered, but may be in future iterations.

## 6  Conclusion

Using models as the basis for agent development allows many of the usual intricacies involved, such as the expert knowledge requirement and complicated design methodologies, to become nearly non-existent. This means that agents can reach a much wider audience, which, considering their abilities and nature, could vastly improve many existing software applications. By further optimizing the way these agents interact and progress, both technical and commercial viability can be achieved.

In this paper, we have detailed our model-driven agent development approach, demonstrating its development, usage, and optimization. Our approach consists of taking an ENFR model, and converting it into an agent through our defined meta-model. The agent can then interpret and select from the operationalizations within this model. Through our approach, this selection process considers the operationalization itself as well as its children. This produces an optimal result with respect to the current state of the agent as well as future states. Our approach is evaluated empirically using an enlarged example existing within a completely dynamic environment. Our approach was required to select the optimal operation plan path through the possible selection set with respect to any random changes that occur. In comparison to other approaches such as static, random and preferential-based, our optimization approach achieved favorable results, performing optimally.

This means that, as well as significantly reducing the complexity involved with agent development, our approach also creates agents which are capable of functionality and optimality that is similar to an agent created through traditional means. Therefore, as well as allowing agent technology to reach a much wider audience, it also enables these audiences to achieve a multitude of typical agent benefits, independent to their development foundations.

Future work for this approach includes the development of a graphical tool which will allow users to draw and label an ENFR model through its interface. This can then be used to directly create the code required for the agent, ready for the user to run, access and manipulate at their discretion. Another future addition is integration with the Prometheus methodology, or the creation of an entirely independent methodology which would allow planning created specifically for these types of agents. This would make their creation much more efficient and handle building the initial ENFR model, which is a requirement of agents created through this approach.

# References

1. Alan, A., Costanza, E., Fischer, J., Ramchurn, S., Rodden, T., Jennings, N.: A field study of human-agent interaction for electricity tariff switching. In: Proceedings of the 2014 International Conference on Autonomous Agents and Multi-agent Systems, pp. 965–972. International Foundation for Autonomous Agents and Multi-agent Systems, South Carolina (2014)
2. Rao, A., Georgeff, M.: Bdi agents: from theory to practice. In: Proceedings of the First International Conference on Multi-Agent Systems, pp. 312–319. The MIT Press, London (1995)
3. Dam, H., Ghose, A.: Automated change impact analysis for agent systems. In: 27th International Conference on Software Maintenance, pp. 33–42. IEEE Press, New York (2011)

4. Winikoff, M.: Implementing commitment-based interactions. In: Proceedings of the 6th International Joint Conference on Autonomous Agents and Multi-Agent Systems, p. 128. Association of Computer Machinery, New York (2007)

5. Nunes, I., Lucena, C., Luck, M.: Bdi4jade: a bdi layer on top of jade. In: 9th International Workshop in Programming Multi-Agent Systems, pp. 88–103. International Foundation for Autonomous Agents and Multi-agent Systems, South Carolina (2011)

6. Pokahr, A., Braubach, L., Lamersdorf, W.: Jadex: a bdi reasoning engine. In: Multi-Agent Programming, pp. 149–174. Springer, Heidelberg (2005)

7. Huget, M.: Agent uml class diagrams revisited. In: Agent Technologies, Infrastructures, Tools, and Applications for E-Services, pp. 49–60. Springer, Heidelberg (2003)

8. Affeck, A., Krishna, A.: Supporting quantitative reasoning of non-functional requirements: a process-oriented approach. In: Proceedings of the International Conference on Software and System Process, pp. 88–92. Australian Computer Society, New York (2012)

9. Burgess, C., Krishna, A.: A process-oriented approach for the optimal satisficing of non-functional requirements. In: Proceedings of the International Conference on Software Process: Trustworthy Software Development Processes, vol. 5543, pp. 293–304. Springer, Heidelberg (2009)

10. Affeck, A., Krishna, A., Achutha, N.: Optimal selection of operationalizations for non-functional requirements. In: Proceedings of the Ninth Asia-Pacific Conference on Conceptual Modelling, vol. 143, pp. 69–78. Australian Computer Society, New York (2014)

11. Nunes, I., Luck, M.: Softgoal-based plan selection in model-driven bdi agents. In: Proceedings of the 2014 International Conference on Autonomous Agents and Multi-agent Systems, pp. 749–756. International Foundation for Autonomous Agents and Multi-agent Systems, South Carolina (2014)

12. Russell, S., Norvig, P.: Artificial Intelligence: A Modern Approach. Prentice Hall, New Jersey (2003)

13. Padgham, L., Winikoff, M.: Prometheus: a methodology for developing intelligent agents. In: Agent-Oriented Software Engineering III, pp. 174–185. Association of Computer Machinery, New York (2003)

# Supporting People to Age-in-Place: Prototyping a Multi-sided Health and Wellbeing Platform in a Living Lab Setting

Wally J.W. Keijzer-Broers, Lucas Florez-Atehortua
and Mark de Reuver

**Abstract** A key challenge elderly people face is the ability to live independently. Losing their everyday independence is a major concern for the elderly, partly because they fear this could lead to an involuntary move to an assisted living facility instead of living independently. Since 2015, the Dutch government encourages their citizens to age-in-place, but at the same time struggles with how to implement new healthcare regulations. To support both government and citizens, we propose a digital platform to match supply and demand in the health and wellbeing domain. Such a platform should not only enable end-users to enhance self-management, but also support them to find solutions for everyday problems related to aging-in-place. To illustrate our Action Design Research we established a Living Lab in a metropolitan area in the Netherlands, and developed a prototype of the proposed platform in a real-life setting.

**Keywords** Smart living · Age-in-place · Living lab · Health and wellbeing platform · Action design research

A prior version of this paper has been published in the ISD2015 Proceedings (http://aisel.aisnet.org/isd2014/proceedings2015/).

W.J.W. Keijzer-Broers (✉) · L. Florez-Atehortua · M. de Reuver
Delft University of Technology, TPM, Delft, The Netherlands
e-mail: w.j.w.keijzer-broers@tudelft.nl

L. Florez-Atehortua
e-mail: l.florezatehortua@student.tudelft.nl

M. de Reuver
e-mail: g.a.dereuver@tudelft.nl

© Springer International Publishing Switzerland 2016
D. Vogel et al. (eds.), *Transforming Healthcare Through Information Systems,*
Lecture Notes in Information Systems and Organisation 17,
DOI 10.1007/978-3-319-30133-4_11

153

# 1  Introduction

The world's population is growing older and, as in many other countries in Europe, the Dutch government is aiming for better integration of health and social care to support elderly people and patients with chronic conditions in the community [1]. An aging population can be explained by the increasing life expectancy due to improved public health and a declining fertility rate. Both trends are expected to continue in the coming decades. Life expectancy at birth will increase globally by ten years, to reach an average of 76 years by 2045–2050. In the same timespan the average global fertility rate will drop to the replacement level. Next to that, the United Nations predict that within thirty years the elderly people will even outnumber children under the age of 15 [2]. One policy to reduce healthcare expenditures is to encourage people to live longer at home (i.e., aging-in-place) [3]. Whilst, most elderly prefer aging-in-place instead of living in an institution [4] and want to maintain a certain quality of life [5], it is a challenge to make this happen. Decrease in cognitive and functional abilities, social exclusion, digital divide as well as time pressure on the caregivers, are typical hurdles. Besides these general difficulties end-users are not aware of what products and services are available to fulfill their needs at a certain point of time. Societal issues related to health, wellbeing and comfort come together in the home-environment of people, but if elderly become more vulnerable, it becomes harder to take responsibility themselves. This requires solidarity from society and especially from voluntary caretakers, friends and family to support active aging [6]. To assist the elderly, considerations need to be given to housing, transportation, social interaction, cultural engagement and activities [7]. Aging-in-place also implies that elderly maintain social connections to the neighborhood and the community, as well as in socio-cultural contexts [8].

Next to that, ICT solutions can help to arrange daily activities in a smarter way. It is not about a smart home per se (i.e., with advanced automated appliances) but how to integrate smart solutions in our daily life. This is related to the concept of smart living defined as an integrated design of our homes and neighborhoods in which functional and non-functional requirements come together in an integrated value-sensitive design. Smart living is related to the quality of life [9] and involves connecting our daily activities at home, along the way, or anywhere else, that can be supported by integrated ICT. Smart Living services are related to the Internet of Things (IOT) that can be interpreted as 'a worldwide network of interconnected objects uniquely addressable, based on standard protocols' [10]. Because of advanced sensor technologies and integrating sensors, devices are transforming into smart objects [11]. Next to that, smart living services can be seen as mediator between providers and customers in the process of value creation [12].

Therefore, we propose a digital platform for health and wellbeing to match supply and demand in the smart living domain. This service platform should not only create awareness among end-users about what services and technologies can help them, but also assist in mediating between (latent) needs and (yet unknown) services.

Ultimately, such a platform should enable end-users to enhance self-management (i.e., independency) by the provision of relevant information and support in matching between different stakeholder groups (i.e., consumers, providers, and government). Eventually the platform has to enhance the quality of life of end-users.

This paper describes the prototyping phase of a health and wellbeing platform in a real-life setting. In Sect. 2 the Action Design Research method is explained and how this is integrated in a Living Lab environment. Section 3 gives insight in the prototyping phase of the health and wellbeing platform. Finally, before the conclusion and future work is discussed, the first usability test of the platform is described in Sect. 4.

## 2  Action Design Research Method

Our research is part of the design research tradition, which is a well-established sub-branch of information systems e.g., [13, 14]. To be more precise, we draw on Action Design Research (ADR) that stresses the relevance circle of Hevner [15] by providing guidance for combining building, intervention and evaluation of an IT artifact in a concerted research effort [16].

Fundamentally, ADR is a study of change and particularly appropriate for our research because: (1) it combines action research (AR) and design research (DR) to generate prescriptive knowledge (2) it is problem-driven and (3) it aims to build design principles based on iterative cycles (see Fig. 1).

The problem formulation in the ADR design mainly adheres to two principles: practice-inspired research and a theory-ingrained artifact. The first principle is

**Fig. 1** ADR design stages and related principles according to Sein et al. [16], p. 41

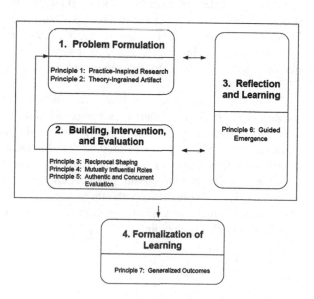

focused on field problems as knowledge-creation opportunities, instead of theoretical puzzles, as in the second principle the artifact can be seen as the carrier of theoretical traces and iterations, based on the theoretical insights that have been obtained.

The second block focuses on the building, intervention, and evaluation (BIE) of the artifact, based on three principles. First, the reciprocal shaping, which means that it should be emphasized on the influences from two domains the IT artifact and the organizational context. Mutually influential roles, refer to the fact that all participants of the ADR team should learn from each other. The principle that is part of the third block: reflection and learning is the guided emergence. This consists of three types of reflections: (1) on the intervention results, (2) the learnings in terms of theories selected, and (3) the evaluation of adherence to the ADR principles. It provides a reflection of the seemingly incongruent perspectives. The last block of ADR is the formalization of learning. It has the principle that the learnings should be abstracted to a class of field problems that should be communicated well.

To reflect on the ADR process and to track the iterative design steps, the action design researcher kept an observation log on a daily basis over the period 2013–2015 amounting up to 700 pages. Next to that, the logbook is used as a scientific record [17] and contains the decision steps related to the design process.

## 2.1  Earlier Research on the Platform

Earlier research on the health and wellbeing platform covered the first stage of the ADR design cycle: 'problem formulation' ([18–21]. In this part of the research we structured the problem and identified the possible solutions to guide the design [22].

As a result of the first design stage, we categorized the suggested features extracted from 70 interviews and 2 focus groups for the health and wellbeing platform before moving to the second stage: the 'Building, Intervention, and Evaluation' phase.

Table 1 illustrates the multiplicity of requirements for platform functions, ranging from basic information exchange towards active recommendations for services and matching, and from pure focus on transactions towards inter-active communication with end-users. Based on the aforementioned features, the platform would be a first mover in the Netherlands to combine and offer; (1) matching between providers of smart living products and services and end-users, (2) finding local activities, (3) connecting with others (e.g., family, caretakers), (4) information about aging-in-place and, (5) integration of successful, existing platforms in the health and wellbeing domain.

**Table 1** List of main features for the platform

|  | Domestic | Health | Wellbeing |
|---|---|---|---|
| Products | Security<br>Home automation | Nursing aids | Entertainment<br>Comfort products |
| Services | Renovation<br>(i.e., installer)<br>Maintenance<br>(i.e., gardner) | Personal care<br>Health care | Comfort services (i.e., grocery,<br>cooking, housekeeping) |
| Local activities | Every day<br>activities<br>Education | Daycare<br>Care related<br>activities | Sports and entertainment<br>Cultural<br>In/outdoor activities |
| Contacts | Family<br>Friends | Patient bonds<br>Health care | Elderly bonds<br>Municipality |
| Information aging<br>in place | Advisors<br>Renovators | Municipality | Advisors<br>Caregivers |
| Integration<br>existing platforms | Radio and<br>broadcasting<br>Restaurants and<br>takeaway | Governmental | Caregivers<br>Volunteers |

## 2.2 Living Lab Setting

To enter the stage of 'Building, intervention, and evaluation' we moved from a pure academic environment to a Living Lab setting. The Living Lab approach represents a research methodology for sensing, prototyping, and validating complex solutions in real-life contexts. Studying behavior in a real-life context allows researchers to gain a better understanding of how the creation of artifacts fit into the complexity of daily life [23]. Living Labs thus can be considered as user-centric environments providing open collaborative innovation. For a successful societal deployment of the proposed platform we needed to address end-users' as well as external stakeholder needs in concert. Feedback from end-users in an early stage of the technology development phase, on elements like relevance and usability are crucial to give a boost to both utilization and delivered value of the application [24]. Understanding the (potential) user can help minimizing risks of a technology introduction. For this reason potential end-users were included in the Living Lab from the start.

To acquire commitment from stakeholders to enter a Living Lab required a lot of effort and resilience of the ADR team. Healthcare related systems are extremely complex and it takes a lot of time to gain understanding, especially when there is no subsidy or financial compensation involved related to the stakeholders' efforts. After several attempts and initial failures related to time, money and priority constraints, we managed to assemble a consortium with multiple stakeholders from eight different disciplines (i.e., municipality, multinationals, SMEs and end-users) that committed itself to the Living Lab. Important drivers for the stakeholders to invest in this pilot were: (1) market access to the health and care domain (2) competitive advantage and (3) business opportunities [23].

Our Living Lab can be described as a Quadruple Helix: a co-operation between large and small to medium size enterprises, the university, public organizations and end-users [25]. In most Living Labs end-users are often consulted 'after the arrow has left the bow', but there are clear benefits to the inclusion of, for instance, citizens in a preliminary stage of the design [26, 27].

The focus of our public sector-centered Living Lab is on the development of public services, so that the municipality can function better and offer new and better products and services to the citizens. To do so, we incorporated user-centered design (UCD), an approach that involves end-users (i.e., the elderly and caretakers) throughout the development process, to ensure that the proposed platform technology meets their needs.

## 2.3  Building Intervention and Evaluation Phase

The second stage of ADR uses the problem framing and theoretical premises adopted in stage one carried out as an iterative process in a Living Lab setting. This phase interweaves the Building of the IT artifact, the Intervention in a real-life setting and the Evaluation of the IT artifact (BIE) (Fig. 2).

During the first BIE iteration, the ADR team challenges participants' existing ideas (i.e., end-users) and assumptions about the platform's specific use context in order to create an alpha version of the prototype.

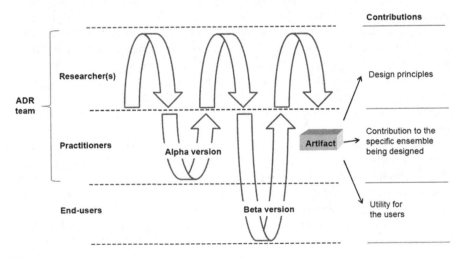

**Fig. 2** BIE iterations according to Sein et al. [16], p. 43

# 3 Building the Alpha Version of the Prototype

In order to track real-time problems during the design process we are using the agile scrum method based on flexibility, adaptability and productivity [28].

As a first step, the ADR team elaborated on the main features (i.e., marketplace products and services, contacts, local activities, information exchange and the integration of existing platforms) for the prototype (see Sect. 2.1) and translated these features into a navigation map from an end-user perspective (Fig. 3).

Based on the main features, the Alpha version of the platform captures basically three core functionalities: (1) a social environment for local activities and contacts,

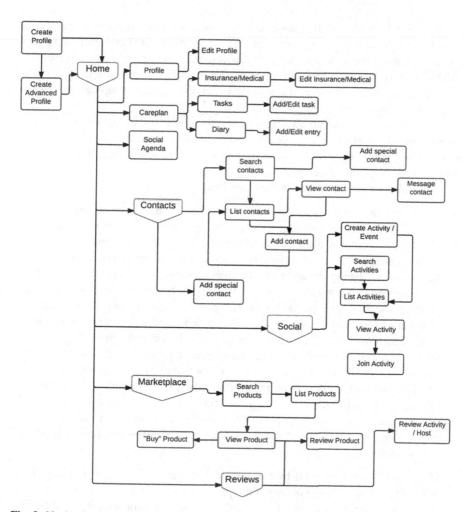

**Fig. 3** Navigation map of the alpha version of the platform

(2) a marketplace for smart living products and services with reviews, and (3) a health and wellbeing profile which can be extended with a personal Care Plan.

The rationale behind the Care Plan is that people themselves can be the center of action-taking related to health and wellbeing, such as measuring, tracking, experimenting and engaging in interventions, treatments, and activities. A Care Plan can contribute to an increased level of information flow, transparency, customization, collaboration, and responsibility-taking aspects from the end-user perspective.

## 3.1 Building the Mockups

As a second step, the ADR team elaborated further on the suggested features to visually represent them in mockups from the perspective of the end-user (see Fig. 4 for a mockup of the Care Plan). Several user-centric design principles were considered in this effort such as visual hierarchy, simplicity, and usage of familiar patterns from successful IT artifacts (e.g., Facebook, google calendar) during the design of the mockups.

Figure 4 is the mockup that represents the view of an informal caretaker responsible for an older person (i.e., Annie). This is illustrated in the top bar of the mockup where it is shown on whose profile the user is acting, self (My home) or someone else's (Annie's home).

There are five key elements in the Care Plan:

- The left menu gives access to the three main features earlier identified as requirements, such as contacts, activities and smart living products and services.
- The agenda contains the tasks assigned to the user (i.e., Annie) given by a doctor, caretaker or relative (or any other authorized user) related to Annie's health and wellbeing. In addition, the agenda contains activities/events, which are occasions that Annie (or someone else on her behalf) has voluntarily joined (through the Activities option on the left menu) as part of her social agenda.
- The diary keeps a record of events, observations, and experiences of Annie so others can have a traceable log of Annie's health and wellbeing.
- Insurance and medical info contains the insurance policy file of Annie and other medical information that is important for Annie and those surrounding her.
- The bottom notification section; this reminds the user to complete the profile (so relevant social activities can be suggested for Annie) and to review products and services acquired (in order to present the feedback to other users and to reduce the customer's perception of risk with the platform when purchasing products and services).

The Care Plan can be used by the end-user, or shared with relatives, a district nurse or even a care broker, but only if the profile owner allows this. In addition, the Care Plan is key in our design for user engagement and adoption; it is a differentiator in terms of meeting the needs of potential users in the context of health and

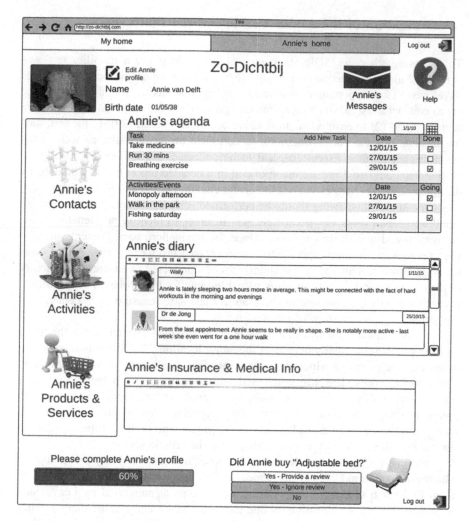

**Fig. 4** Mockup of the care plan

wellbeing. In other words, this functionality allows efficient handling of information for those involved in the care of others.

The proposed platform is a multi-sided platform offering services to individuals and to providers who offer services to the individuals. Such platforms require special attention to privacy because each transaction within the platform is somehow related to personal data of the individual. The platform will be compliant with privacy-by-design principles throughout all the development phases and the entire lifecycle. Consideration of appropriate use of existing Privacy Enhancing Technologies (PETs), as well as the EU Data Protection Directive (Directive 95/46/EC) will be made.

# 4  Evaluation of the Alpha Version of the Platform

To assess whether the ADR team was on the right track, a usability test was conducted almost immediately after the first clickable model of the platform was developed. Two important considerations when conducting usability testing are (1) to conduct a test in which representative participants interact with representative scenarios and (2) to ensure that an iterative approach is used [29]. In the test, data on the time that the participants took to complete the given tasks, as well as the satisfaction with their experience, had to be collected. These data are both quantitative and qualitative and are incorporated in a detailed report that can be used by designers to make changes and test the artifact again. Leavitt and Shneiderman [29] suggest that usability testing should be performed early in the design process with a small number of users (approximately six) in order to identify problems with the navigation and overall design issues. Once the navigation, basic content, and display features are in place, quantitative performance testing (e.g., measuring time, wrong pathways, failure to find content) can be conducted to ensure that usability objectives are met. Besides providing valuable input for the evolution of the artifact towards a usable tool, the role of the usability test is to measure the acceptance of the artifact in an early stage of the design.

The first usability test was in a controlled environment, which means the tester and the participants were gathered in the same location. The test was intended to determine the extent to which the user's interface facilitates the user's ability to complete key tasks. This was conducted with a group of six potential end-users (i.e., elderly, voluntary caretakers and professional caretakers) who were asked to complete a series of tasks with an end goal. Sessions were recorded and minutes were taken to identify critical areas for improvement of the artifact. Figure 5 summarizes the usability test tasks along with the criteria set.

These tasks are related to the three functionalities described in the mockup for which a clickable model was developed in this first iteration. Our benchmarking norm is 5 out 6 successful tasks by the participants as suggested by Leavitt and Shneiderman [29]. As a result only one task ('Create an entry in the diary') didn't fulfill the completion criteria, and two ('Create an entry in the diary' and 'Join activity') the time criteria. The diary concept/functionality in the artifact was not clear for everyone and needs to be revised and enhanced; participants were unfamiliar with the type of text input that we offered.

In a post-test survey participants were asked whether they would use/recommend the platform as well as their satisfaction with their experience; all the participants (6/6) agreed that they would use or recommend the platform if available and 4 out of 6 participants rated 4 or 5 in a scale of 1–5 the user experience of the artifact. The prototype tested was a simple HTML model with no efforts on visual design as yet. Participants also provided qualitative input during the usability test. Font and images size, simplicity and structure of the artifact were praised, whereas specific functionalities like the diary were suggested for improvement.

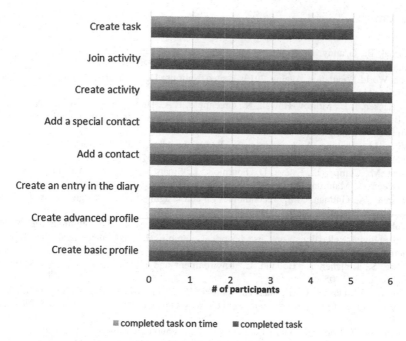

**Fig. 5** Usability test tasks and criteria (N = 6)

## 5 Discussion and Conclusions

Early acceptance of the platform is critical in this research; therefore the results given by the usability test suggest that the right steps are being taken during the design stage. Using familiar patterns when designing a prototype helps potential users to feel more acquainted with the artifact. Preparing a clickable interactive model for a usability test requires far less effort compared to when a fully functional artifact is provided. However, we consider that the effects of testing could be comparable. Although the participants are not provided yet with a full experience, the usability test can be designed in a way that really evaluates critical elements of the artifact based on specific tasks and goals given to the participants as in a controlled setting, creating the feeling of a finalized artifact. Therefore, the approach taken in this iteration step, for the evaluation of the design of the platform, is also suggested for the next iterations. Based on the recommendations of the first testers, we included the mock-up of the design in a large-scale survey (i.e., elderly and informal caretakers) for further data gathering on the subject. In parallel with the data-analysis of the survey, field tests of the clickable model of the platform are foreseen with different groups of informal caretakers, district nurses and potential end-users (age group 55–75). These evaluation moments, that ensure effective participation of end-users, are part of the iterative design steps of the overall ADR project.

# References

1. Rechel, B., Grundy, E., Robine, J.M., Cylus, J., Mackenbach, J.P., Knai, C., McKee, M.: Ageing in the European Union. Lancet **381**, 1312–1322 (2013)
2. UN: World Population Ageing 2013. United Nations, Department of Economic and Social Affairs, Population Division (2013)
3. Carstensen, L.L., Morrow-Howell, N., Greenfield, E.A., Hinterlong, J.E., Burr, J.A., Hudson, R.B., Wilson, S.F.: Civic engagement in an older America. The Gerontological Society of America, Washington (2010)
4. Wiles, J.L., Leibing, A., Guberman, N., Reeve, J., Allen, R.E.: The meaning of "ageing in place" to older people. Gerontologist **52**, 357–366 (2011)
5. Chan, M., Campo, E., Esteve, D., Fourniols, J.: Smart homes—current features and future perspectives. Maturitas **64**, 90–97 (2009)
6. Sixsmith, A., Gutman, G.M.: Technologies for active aging. In Technologies for Active Aging New York. Springer, Berlin (2013)
7. Wahl, H.W., Weisman, G.D.: Environmental gerontology at the beginning of the new millennium: Reflections on its historical, empirical, and theoretical development. Gerontologist **43**, 616–627 (2003)
8. Peace, S., Kellaher, L., Holland, C.: Environment and identity in later life. McGraw-Hill International (2005)
9. Giffinger, R., Fertner, C., Kramar, H., Kalasek, R., Pichler-Milanovic, N., Meijers, E.: Smart cities-Ranking of European medium-sized cities. Vienna University of Technology, New York (2007)
10. Vermesan, O., Friess, P.: Internet of things-global technological and societal trends from smart environments and spaces to green ICT. River Publishers, Denmark (2011)
11. Kortuem, G., Kawsar, F., Fitton, D., Sundramoorthy, V.: Smart objects as building blocks for the internet of things. Internet Computing, IEEE **14**, 44–51 (2010)
12. Grönroos, C., Ravald, A.: Service as business logic: implications for value creation and marketing. J. Serv. Manage. **22**, 5–22 (2011)
13. Hevner, A., March, S., Park, J., Ram, S.: Design science in information systems research. MIS Q. **28**, 75–105 (2004)
14. Gregor, S., Jones, D.: The Anatomy of a design theory. J. Assoc. Inf. Syst. **8**, 313–335 (2007)
15. Hevner, A.: A three-cycle view of design science research. Scand. J. Info. Syst. **19**, 87–92 (2007)
16. Sein, M., Henfridsson, O., Purao, S., Rossi, M., Lindgren, R.: Action design research. MIS Q. **35**, 37–56 (2011)
17. Alaszewski, A.: Using diaries for social research. Sage, London (2006)
18. Keijzer-Broers, W., De Reuver, M., Guldemond, N.: Designing a matchmaking platform for smart living services. Inclusive society: health and wellbeing in the community, and care at home, pp. 224–229. Springer Berlin, Heidelberg (2013)
19. Keijzer-Broers, W., Nikayin, F., De Reuver, M.: Main requirements of a health and wellbeing platform: findings from four focus group discussions. In: ACIS 2014. AUT Library, Auckland (2014)
20. Keijzer-Broers, W., De Reuver, M., Guldemond, N.: Designing a multi-sided health and wellbeing platform: Results of a first design cycle. ICOST 2014—Denver, vol. conference proceedings, pp. 3–12. Springer, Berlin (2014)
21. Keijzer-Broers, W., De Reuver, M., Florez Atehortua, L., Guldemond, N.: Developing a health and wellbeing platform in a living lab setting: an action design research study. In: DESRIST
22. Gregor, S.: The nature of theory in information systems. MIS Q. **30**, 611–642 (2006)
23. Niitamo, V.P., Kulkki, S., Eriksson, M., Hribernik, K.A.: Milan. State-of-the-art and good practice in the field of living labs. In Proceedings of the 12th international conference on concurrent enterprising: innovative products and services through collaborative networks (ICE2006), (pp. 26–28, 341–348). Nottingham, Italy (2006)

24. Abras, C., Maloney-Krichmar, D., Preece, J.: User-centered design. Thousand Oaks: Sage Publ. **37**, 445–456 (2004)
25. Arnkil, R., Järvensivu, A., Koski, P., Piirainen, T.: Exploring the quadruple helix. Outlining user-oriented innovation models. Report of Quadruple Helix Research for the CLIQ Project, Tampere: Work Research Centre. University of Tampere, Tampere (2010)
26. Holzer, M., Kloby, K.: Sustaining citizen-driven performance improvement: Models for adoption and issues of sustainability. Innov. J. Publ. Sect. Innov. J. **10**, 521–541 (2005)
27. Brand, R.: The citizen-innovator. Innov. J. **10**, 9–19 (2005)
28. Schwaber, K.: Agile project management with Scrum. Microsoft Press, USA (2004)
29. Leavitt, M.O., Shneiderman, B.: Research-based web design & usability guidelines. US Department of Health and Human Services, USA (2006)

# The Perceived Impact of the Agile Development and Project Management Method Scrum on Team Leadership in Information Systems Development

Karlheinz Kautz, Thomas Heide Johansen and Andreas Uldahl

**Abstract** This research contributes to the body of knowledge in information systems development (ISD) with an empirical investigation in the form of a case study that demonstrates the positive impact of the agile development and project management method Scrum on team leadership in information systems and software development projects. It also provides a useful operationalization of the concept through six identified indicators for team leadership. Despite the fact that the case unit had challenges with the use of Scrum, the indicators identified the areas where the company had managed to exploit the potential of Scrum and its practices with regard to increasing team leadership. The research results are discussed with regard to the existing Scrum literature and briefly related to complex adaptive systems (CAS) as a foundation for ISD and agile development.

**Keywords** Agile development · Scrum

## 1 Introduction

Over the last decade agile information systems and software development (ISD) has received much attention from researchers and practitioners as an approach for dealing with change and the unpredictable and hardly controllable elements of ISD

A prior version of this paper has been published in the ISD2015 Proceedings (http://aisel.aisnet. org/isd2014/proceedings2015/).

K. Kautz (✉)
Faculty of Business, University of Wollongong, Wollongong, Australia
e-mail: kautz@uow.edu.au

T.H. Johansen
Progressive AS, Herlev, Denmark
e-mail: thj@progressive.dk

A. Uldahl
Ernst & Young, Søberg, Denmark
e-mail: Andreas.Uldahl@dk.ey.com

© Springer International Publishing Switzerland 2016
D. Vogel et al. (eds.), *Transforming Healthcare Through Information Systems,*
Lecture Notes in Information Systems and Organisation 17,
DOI 10.1007/978-3-319-30133-4_12

167

in a dynamic environment. While numerous publications claim a positive impact of agile development and in particular Scrum on ISD, very little empirical work exists to verify these claims. The literature review, which was part of the study, uncovered some notable exceptions. To contribute to this body of knowledge we set out to answer two research questions: What impact has the introduction of the agile development and project management method Scrum on ISD? What is the effect of any deviations from the guidelines for Scrum?

The results we present are part of a larger project where we developed a framework for investigating the impact of Scrum [1]. As ISD has long been understood as a social process with an acknowledged importance of social interaction [2–9] we concentrate on one of these concepts, which is explicitly related to social interaction, namely Scrum's impact on team leadership in ISD.

In the remainder of the paper we first briefly introduce Scrum, and describe our theoretical background and the research setting and method. Subsequently we present and discuss our findings against the existing literature on Scrum and relate them to complex adaptive systems (CAS) theory, a theory which is considered to provide a theoretical foundation for ISD [10] and in particular agile development [11]. We finish with some conclusions and an outlook to future research.

## 2  Scrum—An Agile ISD Method

Scrum is an agile ISD method with a strong focus on project management, which was formalized and tested by Schwaber and Sutherland in the mid 1990s [12, 13]. Scrum focuses on an iterative and nimble development process, on transparency, visibility and on a cooperative, collegial leadership style and cooperation in and between the development team and the customers. In Scrum the development team is called the Scrum team. Unlike traditional development projects where analysts, developers and testers are typically separated, Scrum teams are built on an interdisciplinary basis and comprise all these roles in one team preferably in one physical location. This structure, as well as Scrum's focus on self-organization, aims at creating team dynamics and a better understanding of the tasks to be performed jointly.

Internally, the role of the Scrum master will provide leadership, motivate and facilitate the team in line with the Scrum values, practices and development process. The role of the Product owner has the responsibility to represent the project and product externally to other stakeholders and customers and to handle and manage the tasks that appear in the product and release backlogs [12].

A Scrum development process is structured through a product backlog, which is a prioritized list of required business and technical functions of the envisioned product. It might change in line with the customer's new needs. A release backlog is a prioritized subset of the total product backlog and defines the functions to be included in a release. A Scrum, performed in so-called sprints, is a set of development tasks and processes which a Scrum team carries out to achieve a given sprint goal. The length of a sprint is predefined and typically lasts between 5 and 30 calendar days [12]. What needs to be done during a sprint is determined by a prioritized sprint backlog, which is determined together with a sprint goal before the start of each sprint by the team and Scrum master and others, if necessary, at a planning meeting.

Throughout a project a burn down chart shows the amount of work left to do versus time over a given period [13]. In short daily Scrum meetings project members briefly present what they have done during the preceding day, which tasks they take on that day, as well as any challenges and obstacles that might have prevented them from carrying out their work without any solution being discussed. Scrums of Scrums are additional short meetings by the Scrum masters of projects, which consist of several Scrum teams.

At the end of a sprint, a sprint review meeting takes place where the Scrum team, the Product owner, other management, and one or more customer representatives from the customer [12] assess the team's development process and progress in relation to the predefined sprint goal. Finally the Scrum team, the Scrum master and possibly the Product owner hold a meeting, called a retrospective, to secure learning and further improvement in the team where both the process and the product are assessed and discussed by each individual team member.

# 3 Literature Review and Theoretical Background

In our study we were interested in the impact of a specific method, namely Scrum on ISD. Our literature review was therefore focused on that particular approach and not in general on project management methods' or agile methods' impact on ISD. This limited our sources to writings which take their starting point in agile ISD. We combined a concept-centric with an author-based approach [14] and applied backward referencing of sources. Our original search with keywords such as 'impact of Scrum', 'effect of Scrum', 'impact of Scrum implementation', and 'effect of Scrum implementation' primarily in Google, Google Scholar and IEEE sources lead to about 90 sources of which eight dealt more precisely with our research problem. An additional eight sources were identified through backwards referencing. From that literature we derived a number of concepts and for these concepts indicators for the impact of Scrum on ISD processes and projects. The resulting framework consisted of the identified, interrelated concepts team leadership, process transparency, productivity, quality, employee satisfaction, as well as customer satisfaction and a total of 38 indicators, which defined the concepts on a more detailed level. Here we are focusing on Scrum's impact on the concept of team leadership. We have reported and discussed Scrum's positive impact on productivity, quality, and employee satisfaction and its contribution to creating business value elsewhere [15, 16].

Schwaber [13] emphasizes the importance of project and team leadership for ISD projects. In the literature on Scrum the concept of team leadership focuses on role of the Scrum master and to some extent of the Product owner to support the functioning of Scrum teams; this includes the social aspects of project management and how social interaction between the individual team members is balanced against development processes, practices and tools [13, 17, 18]. These authors agree about the Scrum masters' importance to create engagement and working conditions that in a professional environment allow for collegial relationships, cooperation, and creativity. Appelo [18] accentuates that a Scrum master should take care of the developers' wellbeing and address any conflicts in the teams. Teambuilding and reducing internal conflicts in the team is the indicator we locate here. Moe and Dingsøyr [17] and Appelo [18] put forward too that the Scrum master should remove barriers between developers and the Product owner and other teams, stakeholders, and units. They further contend that the role comprises to act as a problem solver, coach, facilitator and guardian and to protect the Scrum team as much as possible from unnecessary disruptions and disturbances, which assists in establishing a setting with uninterrupted workflow and peace to work. Marchenko and Abrahamsson [19] agree to this. We use these sources to investigate the indicator shielding staff and the workflow, and the indicator guarding and reducing external conflicts. Appelo [18] also in particular emphasizes the creation of motivation for the development team as an essential element of the Scrum master's leadership tasks. We use this as our fourth indicator for team leadership. Landaeta et al. [20] highlight the importance of continuous and organizational learning for Scrum projects and the role the Scrum master plays in ensuring that learning for the benefit of the organization and the developers takes place in these projects. We take the degree to which learning is supported by the Scrum master as another indicator for team leadership. A final indicator, providing of technical direction as part of team leadership, was identified through one interview during our pilot study with the case unit manager.

## 4   Research Setting and Method

We chose a case study approach to research the impact of Scrum on ISD processes and projects. The chosen case organization has approximately 40 years of experience in solving IT tasks. It has about 3000 employees, who are involved in the development of administrative and statutory software solutions. The investigated case department falls into the latter category and has 45 employees. Its sole product is a case management system for municipal job centers, which gives administrators the opportunity to work across different platforms. For the development of the system, the department previously followed the traditional waterfall model. In 2011 it launched the implementation of Scrum as the development model. At the time of our investigation, the department had completed three full releases with Scrum. As such, the department had the profile of the unit of analysis we were looking for: an organization that had recently chosen to implement Scrum, and that had previously utilized the waterfall model. With the former model still in their minds we expected the employees to make candid assessments of the impact of Scrum as compared to the past.

As we were not able to make direct measurements of the identified indicators we chose to directly ask respondents about their perceptions of the given concepts. The indicators were therefore transformed into direct interview questions and validated in a pilot study[1] before putting them to the 11 interview partners, who were available for the study. We developed three largely overlapping interview guides for the three stakeholder groups, with six developers as respondents, four respondents in leadership roles such as Scrum master, Product owner or unit managers and one representative from the service department, responsible for customer liaisons. All interviews were recorded, transcribed and handed to the respondents for approval. The results of our analysis were presented to the participants of this study and the case organization at large.

The data collection with standardized interviews allowed collections of qualitative and quantitative data. We first asked the respondents to numerically assess, on a scale from −5 to +5, for each indicator its individual change, improvement or decline, as compared to the situation before the implementation of Scrum and then to evaluate its impact on the concept team leadership. After that quantitative judgment we asked into the reasons for these assessments, which provided rich qualitative data. This combination of data allowed for data and method triangulation to improve the validity of our findings [21]. The subsequent analysis was based on mean values for the quantitative data within each indicator; these were interpreted on the basis of the qualitative opinions. The results were then compared and discussed with regard to published Scrum guidelines, findings from the literature, and related to CAS theory. It is worth pointing out that the numerical element of the collected data should be considered secondary. The interviews were intended to be the primary source to collect qualitative data with a statistical element—and not vice versa. The quantitative data was exclusively used to create an indication and an overview of any specific area.

# 5 Findings

Table 1 summarizes the respondents' assessment of Scrum's impact on team leadership.

## 5.1 Teambuilding and Reduction of Internal Conflicts

The results concerning team building fall into two categories: half of the respondents had assessed this indictor as unchanged (0) on both dimensions, whereas the

---

[1]As stated earlier we identified one additional indicator, which we termed 'providing technical direction' through the pilot study.

**Table 1** Scores for Scrum's impact on team leadership

|  | Improvement | Impact on team leader ship | Range of score for both dimensions |
|---|---|---|---|
| Teambuilding and reduction of internal conflicts | 1.1 | 1.0 | 0–4 |
| Staff shielding and workflow | 2.8 | 2.5 | 1–4 |
| Guarding and reducing external conflicts | 1.1 | 1.4 | −1 to 3 |
| Motivating the team | 1.9 | 1.4 | −1 to 5 |
| Ensuring learning | 1.7 | 1.6 | 0–3 |
| Providing technical direction | 1.0 | 1.0 | 0–4 |

other half saw a significant improvement. A respondent, who belonged to the first group of respondents, stated about the Scrum master's role:

> It is a question of getting the team to work. I'll say there are the same social conflicts than before, some do not go well together, others do; to get all those to work together, I think, that's what the Scrum master gets a bit little closer to.

Others, who had set their assessment to 0 explained that they had not noticed an improvement, but no deterioration either, neither for themselves nor for their colleagues. Some of those, who perceived a clear improvement in settling personal conflicts, credited this to the Scrum masters and their ability to create teams:

> (...) there is a personnel manager, and our Scrum master to go directly to, and there is the product owner, who is not so much in touch with staff. There are clear reporting lines and procedures.
> I think there is less conflict because you sit together with the same people, across the different professions; the mutual understanding of what everyone is doing, increases. I think it's a definite improvement.

These statements were made by the respondents, who considered this indicator improvement highest. The occurrence of fewer social conflicts is attributed to the fact that there is a designated leader staff can go to when a problem comes up. This counteracts the uncontrolled escalation of problems, while simultaneously a new sense of community grows that prevents social conflicts from arising. Thus an overall improvement had been perceived.

## 5.2 Staff Shielding and Workflow

All respondents felt that there had been a positive development of this indicator. Managers' ability to shield their employees from disturbances as an important aspect of and positive impact on the developers' general workflow was emphasized. As one respondent put it

> (...) on a daily basis, if we disregard those special periods, then I would actually say yes, the managers are really good to watch over us, so we are not bothered unless something has to do directly with Scrum, or something which is regarded as very important (...)

In this context, the influence of the clearly defined leadership roles of the Scrum masters and Product owners was also highlighted:

> I think that things got much better, there are some clearly defined roles, well, when there are some obstacles or issues in the team, they are up for discussion every morning, where the Scrum master will say "Well, I'll find that out" or where the Product owner takes it on, the less the team can handle the issue itself. So it has become so much better.

The positive assessment of this indicator and its impact on undisturbed workflow was also ascribed to improved team work as described above.

## 5.3 Guarding and Reducing External Conflicts

Generally, there was a very positive assessment of this indicator, which deals with the managers' ability to protect their teams from conflicts with other units. Yet, some individuals felt that there had been no significant change. One respondent actually thought that there had been a definite deterioration:

> I think there is more conflict now because we develop in one way, and some other departments develop in a very different way. And so conflicts arise, as they cannot put themselves into our situation. Then, it is the manager's task to ensure that conflicts do not reach down to us.

Although this respondent has a negative perception of the situation, he clearly indicates that it is the managers, who take care of that the teams are not drawn into these conflicts. It was stated that conflicts with other units were avoided because the teams under the lead of Scrum masters were more self-organized, had knowledge and resources from the different areas in their team, and had a better understanding of each other's work, which previous had been performed in different units. The managers' guarding skills and the new organization of work in general improved the relationship to other units. A respondent stated

> (...) where one previous sat and waited for a specific group to finish their task, one always started talking negatively about them, blamed them, it was always their fault that we were delayed and so on (...).

The new, dynamic way of working had an impact on the amount of frustration and the number and intensity of conflicts that arose between departments,[2] as these were now resolved by the Scrum masters and their counterpart project managers. The leaders and managers weighted improvement in this area high and they were content with the way conflicts were handled and kept from the teams, but opinion was divided whether they had improved in preventing these conflicts from happening.

## 5.4 Motivating the Team

The respondents perceived a positive development in the leaders' efforts to motivate and its impact on team leadership. One respondent however was quite negative and believed that distractions from the increased number of leaders, who tried to draw on the same resources at the same time reduced motivation, but he provided no evidence for this. In contrast another respondent, who had scored both dimensions of this indicator high, the first dimension scored 5 and the second 4 justified his high scoring with the following statement

> With the 'leader' I think Scrum master right now, and our Scrum master is really, really good to keep the motivation up and to keep us going and to take care of that; it is super cool to sit here and work.

This enthusiastic opinion is based on Scrum's way to handle the leadership role of Scrum master, but also on the individual Scrum masters' own ways to motivate staff. Another respondent supports this

> (...) We celebrate the many small achievements, in contrast to before where up to five months passed from the time we started until we had finished, or 4 months or whatever it was. Now we have many such things. I do not know, I think the management has been on a motivation course; all possible things happen, they hand out candy, they run all sorts of campaigns and slogans, they have theme songs for all the different teams. I think we joke more than usual, even though we are more productive than usual. So it's actually more fun to be here.

This respondent was quite pleased with the way management had chosen to motivate staff. The frequent celebration of milestones due to a reorganization of the work, as well as the small initiatives helped to raise motivation and improved the work days. As a whole, the results for team motivation were positive, both managers and developers, with the mentioned doubt, agreed that they were more motivated and that their motivation had increased.

---

[2]It had also a positive impact on productivity which is however beyond the scope of this paper (see [15]).

## 5.5  Ensuring Learning

All respondents shared a common positive perception of this indicator, but differed in their reasons for their scorings. The respondents' justifications can be divided into three groups: the first group thought that the assurance of learning through team leadership had improved to some degree; the second group felt that an improvement had occurred, but further improvements were needed; the last group perceived the situation as unchanged. A representative of the first group stated

> It is because we are running Scrum and my managers at least have realized that I think it's really exciting, and that I want to learn more and have an aspiration to become a Scrum master myself at one time, and it also means I have been allowed to do new things, and have been allowed to learn things.

For this respondent it was the way in which Scrum was utilised and his aspiration for further professional development, which lead to his positive assessment. A respondent from the second group said

> It's better, it's clearly better, but I do not think that everything that should be picked, actually gets picked up. We mostly look at techniques and workflows, that's what we look at in retrospectives, not so much at everything else, whether it was a good way to develop, or whether there arise errors out of it, or whether we estimate correctly. These are things we do not hear anything about, I do not get any lessons learned from it. I think we have become really good at that, but we also collected lessons learnt before.

This respondent had previously stressed that the retrospective meetings were only used to talk about method, techniques and workflows and not about the developed product. In view of this, he thought that there was still room for improvement. This position was shared by the respondent from the service department, who was even more critical and had a very clear view that to ensure learning and securing lessons learnt, further amendments were needed specifically regarding the coordination and interaction between the development team and the service department. Finally, a respondent from the last group elaborated very succinctly why he perceived the situation as unchanged

> ... the manager's ability to ensure learning. For my part, not existing before, and not existing now.

On this background we conclude that ensuring learning was an area where the majority of respondents agreed that there had been an improvement, but where many also acknowledged that more has to be done.

## 5.6   Providing Technical Direction

In general, the respondents agreed that the situation with regard to technical direction through managers, now the Scrum masters, had not been significantly improved or deteriorated. The following comment exemplified this attitude:

> I'll say 0, for me this has no significance at all, and I do not think it got better or worse, no I do not think so.

Most respondents shared the opinion that technical leadership would not necessarily contribute positively to the way the organization utilized Scrum. One respondent differed from the others and scored the improvement dimension with 2 and its impact with 3. He put forward that only executing technical leadership provided a deeper understanding of what the individual Scrum teams are working with

> (...) It requires that the Scrum master has a more technical understanding, where a traditional project leader might be good to manage and can do some Gantt charts, and that kind of thing, but not necessarily understands the technical things deep down; and that is how it is, but when you have to have things going, you need to understand the challenges that are there.

Another respondent was also quite excited about the increased technical leadership

> Well, from almost nothing, to actually get technical support, so I would say that we are up at a 4. Because there definitely has come a better understanding of the technique and how the world really hangs together, so it's not just plans and diagrams, it is actually also what happens deep down behind the curtain. I think Scrum has helped with this, also because the manager can go to the Scrum meetings, and actually get an idea of what is happening.

Moreover, this respondent argues that the Scrum processes and not the specific managers are the main reasons for the improvement in technical leadership. The two cited respondents raised the mediocre rating for this indicator.

## 6   Summary and Discussion of Results

The investigation of Scrum's impact on team leadership in ISD was part of a larger study, which both developed and applied a comprehensive framework consisting of six related concepts. Although a presentation of the overall result would give a more comprehensive portrait of the method's impact, we have here focused on one of the key concepts. This still provides some valuable insights and where necessary we will relate to the other concepts. As a starting point for our discussion we summarize the results of our analysis of Scrum's impact on team leadership in the case unit:

We found that there had been a positive change in the respondents' perception of all indicators. The first three refer to resolving different types of conflicts and issues.

In relation to personal and individual tensions, the perception was that the Scrum masters had succeeded in reducing disputes and in facilitating in cases of conflicts. The respondents reasoned that this was due to the Scrum masters' explicit focus on team building, the clearer reporting and communication channels in the teams, as well as the growing social ties and stronger cohesion in the development team, which was seen as a consequence of their new physical closeness.

The problem area of workflow interruptions was perceived as the one, which had had the largest improvement. The respondents were delighted that their leaders fulfilled the clearly defined role as problem solvers and were able to shield the teams from any annoying disruptions to their work. With regard to conflicts with stakeholders and other organizational units outside the teams, the opinions were divided. Most respondents had experienced a positive change, but there were some who had felt a decline. The reasons for a perceived improvement were related to the explicit guardian role the Scrum masters had taken on, the increased interdisciplinary collaboration in the teams and its accompanying increasing understanding of differing professional positions as well as the raising degree of self-organization in the teams under stable and strong governance from their Scrum masters, which decreased the necessary contacts to other units.

With regard to team motivation the respondents' answers indicated a noticeable improvement, which was due to several reasons. The Scrum masters were praised for their explicit emphasis on encouraging staff and for their initiatives to frequently celebrate the achievement of goals and milestones. The restructuring of work in multidisciplinary teams as well as its organization in tasks of manageable size and time periods were also provided as motivating elements. Ensuring learning, in contrast, was the indicator within the leadership role concept, where respondents saw most room for improvement, although overall they had felt some enhancement of that indicator based mainly on an increased number of opportunities to capture knowledge for further advancement of the development processes. These were, however, not yet used to their full potential. Finally, the leaders' ability to provide technical leadership also showed a perceived improvement. This was mainly attributed to the Scrum masters' active participation in the development work.

These favorable results are in line with the results for the other concepts and their indicators, which with the exception of customer satisfaction were all very positive [1]. As with all qualitative studies of this kind we of course have to take the danger of positive bias and a respondents' tendency of reporting future expectations rather than stating actual perceptions into account. On this background, we compare our empirical data first with the literature on agile ISD and project management and in particular the identified writings about Scrum. According to these sources, there are a number of areas that impact on team leadership, these are: Scrum master, Scrum team, self-organization, retrospectives and Scrum of Scrums.

The Scrum master naturally plays a critical role in the team leadership concept. The Scrum master has a wide range of responsibilities to perform. The Scrum master's main function is to act as a facilitator for the Scrum team and to support the smooth operation of the Scrum practices. To rise into a successful Scrum master, an ISD professional needs to be able to motivate, to shield and to guard as well as to ensure learning for the Scrum team [12]. In two of these three areas the Scrum masters in the case unit had achieved the desired effect. There was positive advancement of guardianship and undisturbed workflow as well as with the provision and maintenance of motivation of the development teams. This had also a positive impact on the team's productivity [15] and the quality of the resulting products [16]. With regard to ensuring learning, the Scrum masters had been less successful. They had managed to improve the situation, but had not quite reached the potential benefits Scrum practices could contribute to in this area. The Scrum masters had also played a positive role in providing technical leadership. This indicator was not explicitly mentioned in the literature, but identified through our pilot study. This aspect of their leadership role had some significance for the investigated case unit. It led to a more active participation in the development process, which in turn had a positive impact on the decrease of interruptions to the teams' workflow. It resulted in the Scrum masters' improved understanding of the development process and the product under development. We thus found that technical leadership, not as a primary or sole quality, but in interplay with the other characteristics of a Scrum master appears to be an important contributor to the positive impact of leadership and the management of agile ISD projects.

A well-functioning Scrum team composed of members, who represent different professional backgrounds and are co-located so that the individual team members can develop a mutual understanding and get insight into each other's work is important for reducing any individual and personal conflicts in a development team [12]. The team building and motivational measures instigated by the Scrum masters in the case unit had this effect and provide empirical support for the literature and the impact of leadership on the development of a collegial work environment in which conflicts are few and are resolvable.

The degree of self-organization under the leadership of a Scrum master plays a crucial part in the well-functioning of Scrum teams. Self-organization can be so immersed in a Scrum team that the team is experiencing familial conditions in a sense that close and long-term cooperation can create a very specific social atmosphere, which can strengthen the collegiate bonds and increase the team's functionality. This can be positive and negative; positive in terms of better cooperation, but also negative as strong bonds can lead to mutual cover-up and group thinking [12]. The case unit and its Scrum teams had not been quite reached that stage. They did however experience a significant reduction in both internal team conflicts and conflicts with other teams and units, which can be attributed to a functioning self-organization.

The Scrum masters' balanced approach to self-organization met the objective described in the literature to protect and relieve individual team members from certain tasks. It created an environment where the developers were not constantly disturbed in their work. We found empirical evidence that the achieved degree of self-organization supported and increased the Scrum master's abilities to motivate their teams as predicted in the literature. Moreover the case unit's form of self-organization had contributed to break down disciplinary boundaries and supported the development teams' workflows. In a successfully self-organized team, everyone should have insights into the other team members' tasks, while at the same time the Scrum master has a clearly defined role [12]. This means that when there is a need for input from a specific team member, the other team members are not unnecessarily disturbed, as the tasks have been clearly defined, broken down and distributed. If in doubt, the Scrum master is available to facilitate or solve the problem. This had been mostly but not yet been fully achieved as the developers were still interrupted and disturbed in their work and further efforts will be needed to progress. However, one benefit of team leadership had been achieved already: the interruptions had decreased and if at all came from the right person.

Retrospectives established and facilitated by Scrum masters are a means to ensure learning where the project participants can benefit from their success stories and from things, which have not gone quite so well. According to the literature the benefit of retrospectives is largest when the reflection process comprises both the more managerial Scrum processes practices, the actual development work, and the resulting outcomes as parts of the final product as a whole [13]. As the exploitation of retrospectives as an instrument to ensure learning through the Scrum masters and Product owners as part of their leadership in the case unit exclusively focused on the Scrum processes, it did not have the sought after extent of learning. It actually also affected the teams' productivity [15]. In the literature the avoidance of repeating errors is ascribed to retrospectives. In the case unit retrospectives had not yet been applied to their full potential, yet the perception of the respondents had been that the repetition of errors had decreased. This was attributed to the influence that self-organization had because as a consequence of the increased individual developer's responsibility, team members had become more mindful not to repeat the same mistakes [15]. Individual and collective mindfulness have been reported as characteristics of agile development independently of a particular method or agile practice [22]. This supports that the lack of exploiting retrospectives to ensure more learning in the case organization to some extent has been compensated by self-organization and mindfulness.

According to the literature Scrum of Scrums are often used in large, complex development projects, which are organized in several Scrum teams [13]. This Scrum practice aims at ensuring learning across the various teams. In the case unit some participants took part in Scrum of Scrums, but there were no explicit and clear guidelines on how knowledge was to be harvested and transferred to the actual Scrum teams or for their preservation for future projects, ensured by Scrum of Scrum meetings. Thus the case unit did not follow the literature in this area. If the case unit develops such guidelines and sends its representatives to the Scrum of Scrum meetings with a clear assignment to come back with feedback to their team, this most likely will have an effect on ensuring learning across the different Scrum teams in the unit.

Our overall positive assessment of Scrum on the team leadership of agile ISD and project management confirms empirically the expectations and claims, which are made in many of the conceptual and non-academic writings we had identified in our literature review. It also fills a gap in the area of empirical studies of agile software development [23]. In the absence of quantitative data and with no possibility to make direct measurements and collect such data throughout the project it is however built on subjective perceptions.

Nonetheless, on a more theoretical level our study can be related to complex adaptive system (CAS) theory to find support for the positive impact of team leadership on ISD as one outcome of Scrum. CAS theory underpins agile information systems and software development methods [24] such as Scrum and the case unit appears to be rather successful after its transition to Scrum. On this background the above results can be linked to CAS concepts and principles. If ISD, in our case agile development supported by Scrum, is understood as a CAS, certain characteristics of the process are recognized to facilitate good performance, while others inhibit it [10, 25].

A number of concepts are frequently used when applying CAS. These core concepts are intertwined and mutually reinforcing. Within the area of ISD they have summarized and put forward as follows [10, 26]. Interconnected autonomous agents are able to independently determine what action to take, given their perception of their environment; yet, they collectively or individually are responsive to change around them, but not overwhelmed by the generated information flow. Self-organization is the capacity of these agents to evolve into an optimal organized form, which results from their interaction in a disciplined manner within locally defined and followed rules. Co-evolution relates to the fact that a complex adaptive system and/or its parts alter their structures and behaviors in response to their internal interactions and to the interaction with other CAS where adaptation by one system affects the other systems, which leads to reciprocal change where the systems evolve individually, but concertedly. Time pacing indicates that a CAS creates an internal rhythm that drives the momentum of change, which is triggered by the passage of time rather than the occurrence of events; this stops them from changing too often or too quickly. Poise at the edge of time conceptualizes a CAS's attribute of simultaneously being rooted in the present, yet being aware of the future and its balance of engaging exploitation of existing resources and capabilities to ensure current viability with engagement of enough exploration of new opportunities to ensure future viability. Poise at the edge of chaos describes the ability of a CAS to be at the same time stable and unstable; this is the place not only for experimentation and novelty to appear, but also for sufficient structures to avoid disintegration; CAS that are driven to the edge of chaos out-compete systems that are not. The above analysis has provided examples of interacting interconnected autonomous agents, such as the involved Scrum masters and developers, their self-organization as individuals and as project teams, their co-evolution through knowledge sharing and learning from each other, as well as for time pacing in the short development cycles, and for poise at the edge of time and chaos, for instance with regard to uninterrupted workflow, which thus empirically and theoretically lend support to the identified perceived positive impact of Scrum on team leadership in ISD projects and project management in our case setting.

# 7 Contribution and Conclusion

The normative literature on agile ISD [13] postulates the importance of leadership for ISD in general as well as for agile ASD projects and puts forward several ways such leadership should be achieved, but provides little empirical based evidence how and with what effect such leadership is executed in practice. As our contribution we fill this gap and offer empirical based evidence and theoretical backing of how leadership is performed and what its impact is. As such it exceeds a recent conceptual study [27] on how agile practices enable effective teamwork from a shared mental model (SMM) theory perspective. Another study [28] investigates how empowerment as a prerequisite for motivation is enabled through agile practices; but while acknowledging a relation between leadership and motivation, it has explicitly excluded it from this empirical study. There are further empirical studies on what motivates developers in agile development to be more productive [29] and how agile practices contribute to influence motivation [30], and while teamwork and good management are identified as motivators, the focus is on motivation and not on team leadership. This is also valid for a study on how agile practices contribute to building trust [31] which finds that good leadership in agile ISD is based on trust, but does not investigate leadership further. In contrast our study focuses on leadership per se.

While the usual disclaimers for the shortcomings of qualitative research also apply for our study, our work contributes to the body of knowledge in ISD with an empirical investigation that demonstrates the positive impact of the agile development and project management method Scrum on team leadership in ISD and project management and it provides a useful operationalization of the concept through six indicators. Despite the fact that the case unit had challenges with the use of Scrum, the indicators identified the areas where the company had achieved to exploit the potential of Scrum and its practices with regard to improving team leadership and its effects. Through the analysis we found an interesting area where the case unit differed from the Scrum literature's recommendations. The case unit's handling of retrospective meetings only reflected the actual Scrum process and practices, but not the actual development work and the developed product. This put the unit at the risk of missing out on any knowledge, which could contribute positively to future iterations and development projects. Future research should further investigate the relationship between team learning and interaction of autonomous interconnected team members in retrospectives and how team leadership supported through Scrum both supports and improves, but also results from learning.

Although several authors underline the importance of an open organizational culture for agile development [8, 11, 32, 33] and argue that an innovative and open organizational culture is necessary to develop software and manage projects according to agile principles we decided to disregard the concept as such as we assumed that the culture, its elements, the basic assumptions held by all members of that culture, their values and beliefs, and their artifacts and creations [34] and the cultural changes as a result of an implementation of Scrum would have an impact and become visible through the indicators. In other words, for culture as a broad concept we thought it would make more sense to be implicitly investigated through the team leadership indicators. In hindsight the relationship between culture and team leadership in the use of agile methods such as Scrum does however also merit a thorough investigation through future research on its own.

# References

1. Johansen, T., Uldahl, A.: Measuring the impact of the implementation of the project management method Scrum (in Danish). MSc thesis. Copenhagen Business School, Copenhagen, Denmark (2012)
2. Hirschheim, R., Klein, H., Newman, M.: Information systems development as social action: theoretical perspective and practice. OMEGA **19**(6), 587–608 (1991)
3. Newman, M., Robey, D.: A social process model of user-analyst relationships. MIS Q. **16**(2), 249–266 (1992)
4. Hirschheim, R., Klein, H., Lyytinen, K.: Information systems development and data modeling. Conceptual and Philosophical Foundations. Cambridge University Press, Cambridge, UK (1995)
5. Newman, M., Robey, D.: Sequential patterns in information systems development: an application of a social process model. ACM Transac. Inf. Syst. **14**(1), 30–63 (1996)
6. Wastell, D.G.: The fetish of technique: methodology as a social defence. Inf. Syst. J. **6**(1), 25–40 (1996)
7. Truex, D.P., Baskerville, R., Klein, H.: Growing systems in emergent organizations. Commun. ACM **42**(8), 117–123 (1999)
8. Kautz, K., Madsen, S., Nørbjerg, J.: Persistent problems and practices in information systems development. Inf. Syst. J. **17**, 217–239 (2007)
9. Rosenkranz, C. :Information systems development as a social process: a structurational model. In: Proceedings of ICIS 2011. http://aisel.aisnet.org/icis2011/proceedings/humanbehavior/7 (2011)
10. Kautz, K.: Beyond simple classifications: contemporary information systems development projects as complex adaptive systems. In: Proceedings of 33rd ICIS. Orlando, FL, USA (2012)
11. Highsmith, J.: Agile software development ecosystems. Addison-Wesley, Boston, MA, USA (2002)
12. Schwaber, K., Beedle, M.: Agile software development with Scrum. Prentice Hall, Upper Saddle River, USA (2002)
13. Schwaber, K.: Agile project management with Scrum. Microsoft Press, Redmond, Washington, USA (2004)
14. Webster, J., Watson, R.T.: Analyzing the past to prepare for the future: writing a literature review. MIS Q. **26**(2), 13–23 (2002)
15. Kautz, K., Johansen, T., Uldahl, A. 2013: The perceived impact of the agile development and project management method scrum on information systems and software development productivity. In: Proceedings of 24th ACIS. Melbourne, Australia (2013)
16. Kautz, K., Johansen, T., Uldahl, A.: Creating business value through agile project management and information systems development: the perceived impact of scrum. In: Bergvall-Kåreborn, B., Nielsen, P. A. (eds.) Proceedings of the IFIP WG 8.6 working conference on creating value for all through IT. Springer Publishing, Berlin, Germany, pp. 150–165 (2014)

17. Moe, N.B., Dingsøyr, T.: Scrum and team effectiveness: theory and practice. In: Agile processes in software engineering and extreme programming. Springer, Berlin, Germany, pp. 11–20 (2008)
18. Appelo, J.: Management 3.0—leading agile developers, developing agile leaders. Addison-Wesley. Crawfordsville, Indiana, USA (2010)
19. Marchenko, A., Abrahamsson, P.: Scrum in a multiproject environment: an ethnographically-inspired case study on the adoption challenges. In: Proceedings of the AGILE 2008 conference. Toronto, Canada, pp. 15–26 (2008)
20. Landaeta, R., Viscardi, S., Tolk, A.: Strategic management of scrum projects: An organizational learning perspective. In: Proceedings of technology management conference (ITMC). IEEE international. Norfolk, USA (2011)
21. Andersen, I.: The apparent reality (in Danish). Samfundslitteratur Publisher, Frederiksberg, Denmark (2006)
22. Matook, S., Kautz, K.: Mindfulness and agile software development. In: Proceedings of the 19th ACIS. Christchurch, NZ, pp. 638–647 (2008)
23. Dybå, T., Dingsøyr, T.: Empirical studies of agile software development: a systematic review. Inf. Softw. Technol. 50(9–10), 833–859 (2008)
24. Highsmith, J.: Adaptive software development: a collaborative approach to managing complex systems. Dorset House Publishing, New York, USA (2000)
25. Meso, P., Jain, R.: Agile software development: adaptive systems principles and best practices. Inf. Syst. Mgt 23(3), 19–30 (2006)
26. Vidgen, R., Wang, X.: Coevolving systems and the organization of agile software development. Inf. Syst. Res. 20(3), 355–376 (2009)
27. Yu, X., Petter, S.: Understanding agile software development practices using shared mental models theory. Inf. Softw. Technol. 56(8), 911–921 (2014)
28. Tessem, B.: Individual empowerment of agile and non-agile software developers in small teams. Inf. Softw. Technol. 56(8), 873–889 (2014)
29. de O Melo, C., Santana, C., Kon, F.: Developers motivation in agile teams. In: 38th EUROMICRO conference on software engineering and advanced applications. IEEE Computer Society, pp. 376–382 (2012)
30. McHugh, O., Conboy, K., Lang, M.: Using agile practices to influence motivation within it project teams. Scand. J. IS. 23(2), 85–110 (2011)
31. McHugh, O., Conboy K., Lang, M.: Using Agile practices to build trust in an Agile team: a case study. In: Proceedings of the 19th international conference on ISD. Springer, New York, pp. 503–516 (2011)
32. Cockburn, A.: Agile software development. Addison-Wesley, Boston, MA, USA (2001)
33. Robinson, H., Sharp, H.: Organizational culture and XP: three case studies. Agile development conference, IEEE Computer Society. Denver, CO, USA, pp. 49–58 (2005)
34. Schein, E.: Organizational culture and leadership, 3rd edn. Wiley, San Francisco, CA (2004)

# The Roles of Complementary and Supplementary Fit in Predicting Online Brand Community Users' Willingness to Contribute

Xiao-Liang Shen, Yang-Jun Li and Yongqiang Sun

**Abstract** Recently, we have witnessed a shift in the form of brand communities from firm-centric to customer-centric. In particular, the customer-centric approach allows value co-creation in brand communities by involving customers in various activities that bring a product to the market. It is thus interesting and necessary to examine customers' motivations in helping brands and communities grow and succeed. Based on the person-environment fit framework, this study presents an attempt to investigate community users' knowledge contribution in one of the largest brand communities in Mainland China. The results demonstrate that both complementary fit and supplementary fit significantly predict consumers' satisfaction with and their commitment to the community, which in turn leads to willingness to contribute. The findings will contribute to both research and practice by offering a better understanding of the roles of complementary and supplementary fit in promoting online brand community users' knowledge sharing and contribution.

**Keywords** Person-environment fit · Complementary fit · Supplementary fit · Online brand communities · Knowledge contribution

A prior version of this paper has been published in the ISD2015 Proceedings (http://aisel.aisnet.org/isd2014/proceedings2015/).

X.-L. Shen (✉) · Y.-J. Li
Economics and Management School, Wuhan University, Hubei, China
e-mail: xlshen@whu.edu.cn

Y.-J. Li
e-mail: lyon@whu.edu.cn

Y. Sun
School of Information and Management, Wuhan University, Hubei, China
e-mail: sunyq@whu.edu.cn

© Springer International Publishing Switzerland 2016
D. Vogel et al. (eds.), *Transforming Healthcare Through Information Systems*,
Lecture Notes in Information Systems and Organisation 17,
DOI 10.1007/978-3-319-30133-4_13

# 1  Introduction

The rapid development of the Internet has given rise to the booming of virtual communities. In particular, a number of brand leaders, such as Sales force, General Motors, and XiaoMi, are making significant efforts to build their own online communities to cultivate a strong relationship with their customers. These brand communities have the potential to promote the brands to grow and succeed on the one hand, and greatly facilitate customers to engage themselves in brand-marketing activities and value co-creation process, on the other hand. In view of this, some companies invest heavily in their online brand communities to better manage customers' contribution. For example, General Motors recently announced that they would cut $10 million advertising budget on Facebook, and invest $30 million annually to operate their own brand community instead [1]. In this regard, it is necessary and interesting to explore how to effectively leverage customers' value in the online brand communities.

In fact, scholars have shown increasing interests in investigating customers' contribution in online brand communities. Some traditional theories, such as social exchange theory, social identity theory, social influence theory, and social capital theory have been adopted in prior studies to explain the participants' willingness to contribute in the communities [2, 3]. However, most of these studies just focused on examining the separate effects of customer or community on users' contribution, but neglected the joint and synergistic impact from both of them. It is necessary to notice that, customers' contribution is a combined result of all these factors, and customers will continuously evaluate how well the community may fit with their own goals, values, and interests [4, 5]. To fill the research gap, the current study adopts the person-environment fit (P-E fit) framework to examine the joint effects of customers and community on online brand community users' willingness to contribute. P-E fit is a useful and comprehensive framework to investigate the joint impacts of person and environment on personal performance. The framework measures the degree to which congruence between individual and environmental attributes [6].

The current study conceptualizes the P-E fit from two related but distinct elements, one is complementary fit, and the other is supplementary fit [7, 8]. In particular, the complementary fit is modeled as a formative construct, including demand-abilities fit, need-supplies fit, and unique role fit. Supplementary fit is also treated as a formative construct, including value congruence and interpersonal similarity. In this study, we present an attempt to investigate the mechanisms through which both complementary and supplementary fit affect online brand community users' willingness to contribute.

The remainder of this paper is organized as follows. In the next section, an overview of online brand communities and P-E fit literature is provided. The research model and hypotheses are developed is Sect. 3, which is followed by research method and data analysis results. In the last section, a discussion on the key findings and the implications for both research and practice are presented.

# 2 Theoretical Background

## 2.1 Online Brand Community

A brand community is "a specialized, non-geographically bound community, based on a structured set of social relationships among admirers of a brand" [4], brand communities have attracted much academic and practical attention for decades. Online brand communities originally came from "consumption communities" proposed by Boorstin [9]. He developed a model to demonstrate the relationship between customers and the brand in the consumption communities, and the model is viewed as the traditional model of customer-brand relationship. Muñiz and O'Guinn [4] regarded the brand community as a "customer-customer-brand triad" and they focused on the relationships between customers connected with the brand. Based on the "customer-customer-brand triad", Upshaw and Taylor [10] thought that all the brand related stakeholders, such as employees, customers, suppliers, strategic partners, and other stakeholders should be included in the brand community model. Further, McAlexander et al. [11] pointed out that brand communities are customer-centric, and suggested that brand managers should pay more attention to customers' feelings and experiences, rather than the brand or the product.

Online brand communities have become a new idea for brand managers to integrate their customers' contribution. In particular, many online brand communities are founded and managed by customers themselves to express their love and admiration to the brand [4]. For example, most of tasks in the brand communities are performed by members themselves, including answering the questions asked by other members, teaching newer members how to use the products, and educating them about the norms of the community [12]. In addition, brand managers can gather valuable marketing insights by monitoring customers' communication, or discussing with customers directly. In view of this, customers' contribution is able to cover all aspects of the products and services, from product design, marketing activities, to customer relationship management, which gives customers the opportunity to become the source of innovation and the value co-creators [13]. In this regard, academic attention should be paid to investigate the mechanisms of customers' willingness to contribute in the emerging brand communities.

## 2.2 Person-Environment Fit Theory

Person-environment fit means the degree of congruence or match between the characteristics of person and the environment [6]. In particular, the individual attributes include interests, ambitions, values, and preferences, etc., while situational attributes include goals, values, resources, culture, and opportunities, etc. The theory suggests that members' satisfaction and commitment are likely to be affected by the attributes of person and environment in combine, and they will develop strong satisfaction and commitment when these attributes come to be congruent. In this regard, the P-E fit is believed to improve our understanding of customers' contribution from both personal and situational side.

It is well-documented that P-E fit has been applied and empirically tested in a wide variety of research domains, such as knowledge management, organization design, and industrial psychology [14, 15]. In these studies, P-E fit is conceptualized in different ways, such as person-organization fit, person-occupation or person-vacation fit, person-job fit, person-group fit, and person-person fit [6, 15]. Fit is determined by the comparison with components of person and environment [6]. These studies have demonstrated the effects of different types of fits on human attitudes and behaviors, with some special focus on environmental dimensions such as the job, supervisor, and group. In this regard, a unified and integrated view may provide more comprehensive information towards our understandings of P-E fit. In view of this, the current study conceptualizes the P-E fit in an integrative way from two interrelated but dependent paradigms: one is complementary fit, and the other is supplementary fit.

Complementary fit occurs when the resources of person and environment satisfy what the other needs exactly [7], which can be conceptualized into formative constructs according to Jarvis et al. [16], including demand-abilities fit, need-supplies fit, and unique role [17]. In particular, demand-abilities fit focuses on the personal abilities to meet the demands of the community on the personal side, while need-supplies fit emphasizes the resources of the community to satisfy individual needs on the environmental side. Unique role is conceptualized as the persons' unique contribution to the environment [17]. Supplementary fit occurs when the characteristics of both person and environment come to be similar with each other [7], which is subdivided into value congruence and interpersonal similarity [17], also as a formative construct Jarvis et al. [16]. In particular, value congruence concept posits that fit is determined by the congruence between individual and situational goals and values. Interpersonal similarity means the similar demographic and psychographic between members in the organization [17]. These formative structures of complementary and supplementary fit are empirically tested to be valid [17].

In summary, the current study conceptualizes the P-E fit into two related fits with a formative constructs: one is complementary fit, subdivided into need-supplies fit, demand-abilities fit, and unique role; the other is supplementary fit, including value congruence and interpersonal similarity. It thus provides us a comprehensive and succinct framework to study P-E fit. In this regard, it is reasonable to adopt complementary and supplementary fit in the research model, and the outcomes will be considered next.

# 3  Research Model and Hypotheses

Based on the person-environment fit theory, as noted above, the theoretical model is presented in Fig. 1.

As discussed earlier, we identified complementary fit as a formative construct, including need-supplies fit, demand-abilities fit, and unique role. In addition, it is believed that the good complementarities between person and the community will impel customers' satisfaction with and commitment to the focal brand community. In particular, need-supplies fit reflects the resources supplied by the community are able to meet members' needs. Needs-fulfillment theory indicates that a person will become satisfied [18], and have an attachment or a desire to stay in the focal community [19], when their needs are met with the supplies provided by the environment. In view of this, the need-supplies fit is believed to exert positive impacts on customers' satisfaction and commitment. Demand-abilities fit underlines the individuals' abilities to meet the organization's demands. If a person has sufficient abilities to meet the demands of the community, s/he will have active interactions with other members in the community. The abilities are believed to make the interaction to be a good experience for a person, and the helping behavior is likely to result in a good relationship between members. In this regard, members will gain satisfaction and have confidence to stay in the community, once they perceive their abilities to satisfy demands of the community. Unique role refers to the unique contribution a person makes to the environment. When a person is unique in the community, s/he will gain more attention from others, and have an irreplaceable position in the community. The irreplaceability is believed to bring some additional value, such as privilege, preferential treatment, and respect. In addition, the uniqueness is likely to disappear when they leave to other organizations. In view of this, unique role will lead to personal satisfaction and commitment. In summary, we have the following hypotheses:

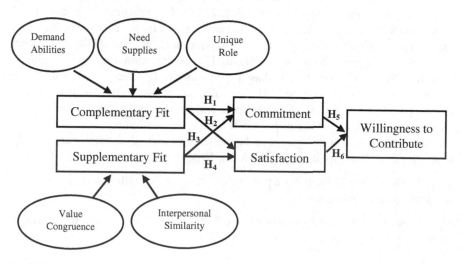

**Fig. 1**  Research model

**Hypothesis 1** Complementary fit has a positive effect on users' commitment to the online brand community.

**Hypothesis 2** Complementary fit has a positive effect on users' satisfaction with the online brand community.

Supplementary fit is subdivided into two interrelated and dependent formative constructs as interpersonal similarity and value congruence. People will find it comfortable to interact with others in a community, where his/her values and goals are advocated by the community as well. This is explained by the fact that the shared values and similar interpersonal characteristics are thought to result in effective communication [20]. In general, since organizational values and goals delineate how to allocate the organizational resources and specify how members should behave, the common values and goals will make it smooth to get resource from the organization [8]. In this regard, customers will be satisfied and committed when they feel consistent with the values and goals of the community. In addition, people are easy to be attracted to others with similar demographic and psychographic characteristics, and then trust them, which reduce uncertainty and improve interpersonal relationships [17]. In this regard, interpersonal similarity is likely to exert positive effects on customers' satisfaction with and commitment to the community. In summary, supplementary fit is thus believed to influence customers' satisfaction and commitment. The hypotheses are proposed in the following:

**Hypothesis 3** Supplementary fit has a positive effect on users' commitment to the online brand community.

**Hypothesis 4** Supplementary fit has a positive effect on users' satisfaction with the online brand community.

As noted above, commitment and satisfaction are identified as the outcomes of P-E fit. Commitment is conceptualized as "a desire to have a continued relation-ship and an effort to ensure its continuance" [21, 22]. In particular, high committed members are believed to care more about the success of the focal communities, and then maybe conduct pro-organizational behavior, such as contributing their own knowledge and experience to the community [21]. Satisfaction refers to individuals' overall sense of well-being based on assessing the environment or environment-related experience [23]. Specially, according to the social exchange theory, people strive for the balance of give and get through social exchange [24]. In view of this, if a participant is satisfied with the community, s/he is likely to reciprocate with his/her knowledge and experience in the online community to help others [3, 24]. Thus, we have the following hypotheses:

**Hypothesis 5** Commitment has a positive effect on users' willingness to contribute in online brand community.

**Hypothesis 6** Satisfaction has a positive effect on users' willingness to contribute in online brand community.

# 4 Research Method

## 4.1 Data Collection

The target population of the study is users who interact with each other in the XiaoMi Community (bbs.xiaomi.cn). The reason why we chose this online brand community is because it is one of the largest and most typical customer-centric online brand communities in Mainland China. An online survey was used, and a total of 480 useful responses were received. Most of the respondents had a bachelor degree (about 70 %), with 37.7 % were aged from 18 to 22 years old. The sample was comprised of 51.3 % of males and 48.7 % of females. In particular, most respondents (85.4 %) reported that they will post on the community per week, and nearly 37.1 % visit the XiaoMi Community more than 6 times each week.

## 4.2 Measurement

In the survey instrument, all the constructs are measured with items adapted from validated measures in prior studies. In particular, P-E fit factors are measured with GEFS items proposed by Beasley et al. [17]. Commitment is measured by items adapted from Liang et al. [22] and Bateman et al. [21]. The items measuring satisfaction are adapted from Bhattacherjec [25]. Willingness to contribute is measured with items adapted from Tong et al. [26]. In addition, seven-point Likert-scale from 1 (strongly disagree) to 7 (strongly agree) was used in the survey. All the items have been slightly modified to fit the specific research context.

# 5 Data Analysis and Results

Smart PLS 2.0. M3 was used in this study to examine the research model. Following the guidelines of two-step analytical procedures, we first examined the measurement and assessed the structural model then. Further, there are differences in assessing the measurement model of formative and reflective constructs.

## 5.1 Measurement Model

To examine the reliability and validity of reflective constructs, construct reliability, convergent validity and discriminant validity were examined in this study. Construct reliability was assessed by testing the composite reliability and the average variance extracted (AVE) [27]. A composite reliability of 0.70 or above

**Table 1** Loadings and cross loadings

| Constructs | CR | AVE | $\alpha$ | Items | COM | SAT | WTC |
|---|---|---|---|---|---|---|---|
| Commitment (COM) | 0.898 | 0.687 | 0.849 | COM1 | **0.850** | 0.402 | 0.425 |
| | | | | COM2 | **0.844** | 0.336 | 0.483 |
| | | | | COM3 | **0.824** | 0.281 | 0.392 |
| | | | | COM4 | **0.798** | 0.298 | 0.435 |
| Satisfaction (SAT) | 0.913 | 0.723 | 0.872 | SAT1 | 0.389 | **0.786** | 0.352 |
| | | | | SAT2 | 0.340 | **0.866** | 0.314 |
| | | | | SAT3 | 0.299 | **0.901** | 0.313 |
| | | | | SAT4 | 0.320 | **0.846** | 0.283 |
| Willingness to Contribute (WTC) | 0.900 | 0.751 | 0.834 | WTC1 | 0.462 | 0.338 | **0.866** |
| | | | | WTC2 | 0.422 | 0.335 | **0.858** |
| | | | | WTC3 | 0.480 | 0.297 | **0.876** |

Note: *CR* composite reliability, *AVE* average variance extracted, $\alpha$ = Cronbach's $\alpha$

and an average variance extracted of more than 0.50 are deemed acceptable [28]. As shown in Table 1, all the measures of reflective constructs exceed the recommended thresholds.

Convergent and discriminant validity were examined using confirmatory factor analysis (CFA). In particular, convergent validity indicates the degree to which the theoretically-related measures are highly correlated with each other, and thus the loadings of all the items in their latent constructs should be higher than 0.7 [28]. Discriminant validity indicates to what degree a given construct differs from other constructs, and thus the item loadings on the intended constructs should be higher than loadings on other constructs [28]. The results in Table 1 depicted a satisfactory convergent and discriminant validity.

In addition, to test the reliability and validity of formative constructs, we condensed the two high-order constructs (e.g., complementary fit and supplementary fit) by using factor scores of the sub-constructs as items of the higher-order construct. The construct validity of formative constructs was assessed by examining the item weights. As shown in Table 2, weights for all items are statistically significant, indicating these items have important and relative contributions to both complementary fit and supplementary fit.

**Table 2** Item weights of formative constructs

| Constructs | Item | Weights | $t$-value |
|---|---|---|---|
| Complementary Fit | CF1 | 0.413 | 37.666 |
| | CF2 | 0.326 | 28.707 |
| | CF3 | 0.447 | 39.096 |
| Supplementary Fit | SF1 | 0.595 | 29.261 |
| | SF2 | 0.610 | 29.770 |

Note: *CF1* demand-abilities fit, *CF2* need-supplies fit, *CF3* unique role
*SF1* value congruence, *SF2* interpersonal similarity

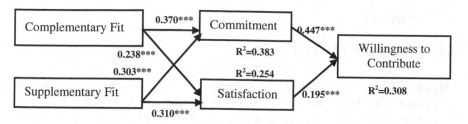

**Fig. 2** Result of PLS Analysis. Note: $*p < 0.05$, $**p < 0.01$, $***p < 0.001$

## 5.2 Structural Model

Figure 2 presents the overall explanatory power, the estimated path coefficients (significant paths are indicated with asterisks), and the associated t-value of the paths. Test of significance of all paths were performed using the bootstrap resampling procedure.

The results of PLS analysis revealed that all hypotheses were supported. Both commitment and satisfaction together explained 30.8 % of the variance in willingness to contribute, with path coefficients at 0.447 and 0.195, respectively. This model also accounted for 38.3 % of the variance in commitment, and 25.4 % of the variance in satisfaction. The results showed that complementary fit has significant impacts on commitment and satisfaction, with path coefficients at 0.370 and 0.238. Supplementary fit also exerts great effect on commitment and satisfaction, with path coefficients at 0.303 and 0.310.

We further examined the mediating effects of community commitment and users' satisfaction on the relationships between P-E fit factors and willingness to contribute in online brand community. Based on the method proposed in Baron and Kenny [29], we have performed the mediating analysis, and as shown in Table 3, the results indicated that both commitment and satisfaction partially mediated the effects of complementary and supplementary fit on community users' willingness to contribute.

**Table 3** Mediating effects of commitment and satisfaction

| IV | M | DV | IV → DV | Mediating effects | | | Results |
|----|---|----|---------|-------------------|---|---|---------|
| | | | | IV → M | IV + M → DV | | |
| | | | | | IV → DV | M → DV | |
| CF | COM | WTC | 0.523*** | 0.580*** | 0.332*** | 0.333*** | Partial |
| CF | SAT | WTC | 0.523*** | 0.451*** | 0.446*** | 0.172*** | Partial |
| SF | COM | WTC | 0.463*** | 0.564*** | 0.254*** | 0.382*** | Partial |
| SF | SAT | WTC | 0.463*** | 0.474*** | 0.368*** | 0.201*** | Partial |

Note: 1. *IV* independent variable, *M* mediator, *DV* dependent variable
2. $*p < 0.05$, $**p < 0.01$, $***p < 0.001$

# 6 Discussion

## 6.1 Discussion of Key Findings

This study focuses on the knowledge contribution in the customer-centric online brand community from the perspective of person-environment fit theory. The result suggests that both complementary and supplementary fit exert significant effects on users' commitment and satisfaction, which in turn influence their willingness to contribute. In addition, this study also investigates the mediating role of both satisfaction and commitment on the relationships between person-environment fit and users' willingness to contribute. The results demonstrate the partial mediating effects of satisfaction and commitment in the relationships. In this regard, our findings support the main idea that community members with high person-environment fit perceptions are more likely to share and contribute, by means of increasing their satisfaction with and commitment to the focal community.

## 6.2 Limitations and Future Research

This study has highlighted the mechanism through which person-environment fit may affect participants' contribution intention in the customer-centric brand community. Before we discussed the implications for both research and practice, limitations of this study will be explored.

First of all, our data was collected using an online survey method, which reflects respondents' subjective perceptions towards the investigated questions. Subjective data has some inherent drawbacks that is hard to be avoided in survey. In this regard, objective data such as archival data or even brain activity data may help to provide additional insights to the specific research domain being explored. Therefore, we recommend future research to obtain and utilize objective performance data to examine participants' behavior in online brand community.

Second, although we have adopted random sampling method in this study to reduce response bias, the self-selected nature of survey method may also result in the bias problems. In this regard, we believe future research could integrate some other research methodologies, such as social network analysis or quasi-experiment, to balance the active and the inactive respondents.

Third, community commitment and satisfaction have explained 30.8 % of the variance in users' willingness to contribute in online brand community, and partially mediated the relationships between P-E fit and contribution intention. It is clear that the two factors play some important roles in understanding community users' pro-social behavior. However, in order to keep the model simple and controllable, some other important variables, such as engagement and trust, are omitted in this study. Future research should nonetheless extend this line of research, and further investigate the influencing mechanism of complementary and supplementary fit on willingness to contribute in online brand community.

Last but not the least, with the booming of online brand communities and the significant role of customers in value co-creation process, academic research should pay more attention to customers' decision making differences in firm-centric brand community and customer-centric brand community, with a specific focus on person-environment fit. Due to the space limit, we will leave this work for future research.

## 6.3  Theoretical and Practical Implications

The current study will contribute to the existing research in following ways. First, the current study focuses on the members' willingness to contribution in the context of XiaoMi Community, one of the most typical customer-centric brand communities in Mainland China. It is generally accepted that the customer-centric approach has facilitated the value co-creation and brand marketing greatly. In this regard, academic attention to such a brand community thus will highlight the value of customers in the brand community and further improve our understanding of this emerging phenomenon.

Second, we conceptualize the person-environment fit as complementary fit and supplementary fit, regardless of the specific situation such as person-organization fit, person-job fit, and person-group fit. In addition, the study further develops and empirically tests the formative structures of complementary and supplementary fit, based on the GPES proposed by Beasley et al. [17]. It thus simplifies the construction of person-environment fit in the previous research, and provides a comprehensive approach to understanding person-environment fit for the future research.

Third, the current study adopts the person-environment fit framework to investigate the customers' motivation behind knowledge contribution in the community. It is believed that users' commitment and satisfaction, and further their behavior in the online community will be influenced by the characteristics of both person and environment. In this regard, it is necessary and reasonable to investigate the joint effects of person and environment on customers' satisfaction and commitment, which shape the relationships between P-E fit and customers' willingness to contribute. Thus, this study enhances our theoretical understanding of knowledge contribution based on the person-environment fit framework.

On the other hand, this study also is available for useful suggestions for the brand managers. Since the customer-centric approach plays a key role in the success of brand community, brand managers should try to maintain a good relationship with customers, and attract customers to engage in the brand community activities. In addition, the congruence between customers and community should be concerned more. That is because it exerts significant effects on customers' commitment to and satisfaction with the focal community, which are believed to facilitate online community users' willingness to contribute. In this regard, the brand managers should pay more attention to the customers' demands and abilities, and further their values and preferences.

# 7 Conclusion

This study shows that person-environment fit theory is a valid framework to understand the knowledge contribution in the customer-centric brand community. By surfacing the motivation of participants to contribute in the community, we find the fit between participants and community has a significant effect on the satisfaction and commitment, which in turn influence behaviors of participants in the customer-centric brand community. In the light of the customer-centric brand community, we hope our findings will provide guidance to others aimed at extending the person-environment fit theory in the virtual community.

**Acknowledgements** The work described in this paper was partially supported by the Humanities and Social Sciences Foundation of the Ministry of Education, China (Grant No.13YJC630132) and the National Natural Science Foundation of China (Grant Nos.71301125, 71231007), without which the timely production of the current publication would not have been feasible.

# References

1. Barkholz, D.: Net worth: GM's Paid-ad pullback highlights a key question for auto marketers: can facebook sell cars? Automot. News (6517) (2012)
2. Chai, S., Kim, M.: A socio-technical approach to knowledge contribution behavior: an empirical investigation of social networking sites users. Int. J. Inf. Manage. 32(2), 118–126 (2012)
3. Chiu, C.M., Hsu, M.H., Wang, E.T.: Understanding knowledge sharing in virtual communities: an integration of social capital and social cognitive theories. Decis. Support Syst. 42(3), 1872–1888 (2006)
4. Muñiz Jr, A.M., O'Guinn, T.C.: Brand community. J. Consum. Res. 27(4), 412–432 (2001)
5. Cable, D.M., Edwards, J.R.: Complementary and supplementary fit: a theoretical and empirical integration. J. Appl. Psych. 89(5), 822–834 (2004)
6. Kristof-Brown, A.L., Zimmerman, R.D., Johnson, E.C.: Consequences of individuals' fit at work: a meta-analysis of person-job, person-organization, person-group, and person-supervisor fit. Pers. Psychol. 58(2), 281–342 (2005)
7. Muchinsky, P.M., Monahan, C.J.: What is person-environment congruence? supplementary versus complementary models of fit. J. Vocat. Behav. 31(3), 268–277 (1987)
8. Kalliath, T.J., Bluedorn, A.C., Strube, M.J.: A test of value congruence effects. J. Organ. Behav. 20(7), 1175–1198 (1999)
9. Boorstin, D.: Consumption communities. Boorstin D. J The Americans: The democratic experience, Pt. II: 89–164 Vintage Books, New York (1974)
10. Upshaw, L., Taylor, E.: Building business by building a masterbrand. J. Brand Manage. 8(6), 417–426 (2001)
11. McAlexander, J.H., Schouten, J.W., Koenig, H.F.: Building brand community. J. Mark. 66(1), 38–54 (2002)
12. Almeida, S.O.d., Mazzon, J.A., Dholakia, U., Müller Neto, H.: Participant diversity and expressive freedom in firm-managed and customer-managed brand communities. Braz. Adm. Rev. 10(2), 195–218 (2013)
13. Sawhney, M., Balasubramanian, S., Krishnan, V.V.: Creating growth with services. MIT Sloan Manage. Rev. 45(2), 34–44 (2003)

14. Pee, L.G.: The effects of person-environment fit on employees' knowledge contribution. In: Proceedings of the 33rd International Conference on Information Systems (ICIS-33), 16–19, Orlando Florida, USA December (2012)
15. Edwards, I.R., Shipp, A.I.: The relationship between person-environment fit and outcomes: an integrative perspectives on organizational fit. In: Ostroff, C., Judge, T.A. (eds.) Perspectives on Organizational Fit, pp. 209–258. Jossey-Bass, San Francisco (2007)
16. Jarvis, C.B., MacKenzie, S.B., Podsakoff, P.M.: A critical review of construct indicators and measurement model misspecification in marketing and consumer research. J. Consum. Res. **30** (2), 199–218 (2003)
17. Beasley, C.R., Jason, L.A., Miller, S.A.: The general environment fit scale: a factor analysis and test of convergent construct validity. Am. J. Community Psychol. **50**(1–2), 64–76 (2012)
18. Cable, D.M., DeRue, D.S.: The convergent and discriminant validity of subjective fit perceptions. J. Appl. Psych. **87**(5), 875–884 (2002)
19. Meyer, J.P., Allen, N.J.: A three-component conceptualization of organizational commitment. Hum. Resour. Manage. Rev. **1**(1), 61–89 (1991)
20. O' Reilly, C.A., Chatman, J., Caldwell, D.F.: People and organizational culture: a profile comparison approach to assessing person-organization fit. Acad. Manage. J. **34**(3), 487–516 (1991)
21. Bateman, P.J., Gray, P.H., Butler, B.S.: Research note-the impact of community commitment on participation in online communities. Inf. Syst. Res. **22**(4), 841–854 (2011)
22. Liang, T.P., Ho, Y.T., Li, Y.W., Turban, E.: What drives social commerce: the role of social support and relationship quality. Intl. J. Electron. Commer. **16**(2), 69–90 (2011)
23. Locke, E.A.: The motivation sequence, the motivation hub, and the motivation core. Organ. Behav. Hum. Decis. Process. **50**(2), 288–299 (1991)
24. Emerson, R.M.: Social Exchange Theory. Ann. Rev. Soc. **2**(1), 335–362 (1976)
25. Bhattacherjee, A.: Understanding information systems continuance: an expectation-confirmation model. MIS Q. **25**(3), 351–370 (2001)
26. Tong, Y., Wang, X., Tan, C.H., Teo, H.H.: An empirical study of information contribution to online feedback systems: a motivation perspective. Inf. Manage. **50**(7), 562–570 (2013)
27. Hair, J.F., Black, W.C., Babin, B.J., Anderson, R.E., Tatham, R.L.: Multivariate data analysis: Pearson Prentice Hall Upper Saddle River, NJ (2006)
28. Fornell, C., Larcker, D.F.: Evaluating structural equation models with unobservable variables and measurement error. J. Mark. Res. **18**(1), 39–50 (1981)
29. Baron, R.M., Kenny, D.A.: The moderator-mediator variable distinction in social psychological research: conceptual, strategic, and statistical considerations. J. Pers. Soc. Psychol. **51**(6), 1173–1182 (1986)

# Understanding Digital Inequality: Studying the Use of Mobile Business Supporting Features in China

Shang Gao and Xuemei Zhang

**Abstract** Today, the Internet has become an essential part of peoples' daily lives. With the advance of Internet technology, the phenomenon of digital inequality has received substantial attention. This study extended research on digital inequality to the field of mobile business. The paper aimed to understand the impact of digital inequality in the use of mobile business supporting features in China. To address this, an empirical study with 258 subjects was carried out. The results indicated that perceived ease of use had a significant positive effect on the use of mobile business supporting features, while perceived risk had a significant negative effect on the use of mobile business supporting features. Furthermore, this study also revealed that socio-economically disadvantaged individuals were more likely to be influenced by perceived risks, while socio-economically advantaged individuals were more likely to be influenced by the utilitarian motivations.

**Keywords** Digital inequality · Mobile business · TAM

## 1 Introduction

Today, the Internet has become an essential part of many peoples' daily lives. The Internet is able to bring many potential values to the society, such as creating new value, increasing social wealth and enhance social happiness. However, many

---

A prior version of this paper has been published in the ISD2015 Proceedings (http://aisel.aisnet.org/isd2014/proceedings2015/).

---

S. Gao (✉)
Department of Computer and Information Science, Norwegian University
of Science and Technology, Trondheim, Norway
e-mail: shanggao@idi.ntnu.no

X. Zhang
School of Business Administration, Zhongnan University of Economics and Law,
Wuhan, China
e-mail: xuemo123@foxmail.com

© Springer International Publishing Switzerland 2016
D. Vogel et al. (eds.), *Transforming Healthcare Through Information Systems*,
Lecture Notes in Information Systems and Organisation 17,
DOI 10.1007/978-3-319-30133-4_14

scholars have noticed the impact of digital inequality on the various applications on the Internet [1]. The research on digital inequality in the use of e-business applications has received increasing attention. For instance, Buhtz et al. have studied the second-order digital inequality in the use of e-business in the US [2], and presented a conceptualized research framework for digital inequality study in the context of e-business.

Advanced mobile technologies offer opportunities to support mobile business work processes in real-time irrespective of time and location of users. However, to our knowledge, the research on the impact of digital inequality in the use of mobile business supporting features is relatively absence. According to the 2014 annual report from China Internet Network Information Center (CNNIC), the scale of China's Internet users has reached 649 million at the end of 2014 and the percentage of those using mobile phones to access the web has jumped from 81 % in 2013 to 86 % at the end of 2014. The mobile business is booming rapidly in China. China, as a fast-growing developing country, has the largest number of mobile phone users all over the world. Mobile business is booming in China. It is interesting to examine how mobile business supporting features are used by different users in China. Therefore, we aimed to understand the impact of digital inequality in the use of mobile business supporting features in China in this study.

By using mobile business supporting features like group purchasing, price comparison sites or taxi booking, consumer can easily search products and services and compare their price on mobile devices. This is different from the traditional market, in which product availability, position, and pricing are highly associated with the place of residence. For instance, mobile coupons are means by which individuals can shop cheaper on their mobile devices than in the traditional market. But not everyone is able to receive economic gains from the use of mobile business supporting features. People with different Internet skills, level of education and socio-economic status may behave differently when using mobile business supporting features. Digital inequality always existed among users of mobile business supporting features. Concerning the theme of mobile business, first-order digital inequality refers to the inequality of mobile business applications access, while the second-order digital inequality refers to different manners of using mobile business applications. The objective of this research is to explore the influence of an individual socio-economic status on the use of mobile business supporting features.

The remainder of this paper is organized as follows: the theoretical background is provided in Sect. 2. Section 3 proposes the research model and hypothesis. This is followed by the presentation of the research method and research results in Sect. 4. The findings of this research are discussed in Sect. 5. Section 6 presents the implications of this research. Section 7 concludes this research.

## 2 Background

### 2.1 Digital Inequality

The term digital inequality often referred to the gaps in access to a computer and Internet access. DiMaggio et al. defined digital inequality as the difference between individuals regarding their access to, and ability to use, information and communication technology [3]. Previous research has focused on the first-order digital inequality [4], which meant the access to information communication technology and its sociological implications, such as, the lack of online education opportunities [5]. Recent research has paid attention to the second-order digital inequality [6]: rather than exploring whether individuals use ICT or not, the study focuses on examining differences in how people use ICT to create opportunities for themselves. The second-order digital inequality tends to focus on the different ways how people use ICT depending on their socio-economic status.

Previous research also paid increasing attention to the phenomenon of digital inequality in various themes (e.g., e-business, e-government). Mossberger et al. [7] have proposed three kinds of performance of digital inequality: firstly, the differences in access and operation of information technology among people, secondly, the differences in economic opportunities resulting from people's inability to participate in Internet-based education, training and lack of hiring opportunities, thirdly, the difference in democracy caused by inability to participate in e-government. Furthermore, scholars have researched variations in Internet skill among different people [8] and digital inequality in the use of electronic government [9]. Last but not least, Buhtz et al. [2] explored second-order digital inequality within the context of e-commerce in the US.

### 2.2 Socio-Economic Status

Digital inequality has been studied in different dimensions including gender, race and age [10, 11]. Furthermore, income and the level of education have been identified as another two key dimensions to reflect the socio-economic difference between individuals [12]. For example, Van Deursen and Van Dijk [13] studied the Internet skill of the Dutch and revealed that lower education would lead to lower Internet skills. In the recent study, Buhtz et al. [2] investigated the relationship between socio-economic status and the use of E-business supporting features and found that the socio-economically advantaged individuals use e-business more effectively than the socio-economically disadvantaged individuals with respect to e-business supporting features.

## 2.3  Technology Diffusion Theory

The Technology Acceptance Model (TAM) was the most influential model to investigate the acceptance of information technology [14]. Perceived ease of use and perceived usefulness were two factors in the original TAM model [14]. The main notion in TAM is that peoples' attitudes toward a technology are shaped by their beliefs about the attributes of this technology, which in turn influence peoples' intentions to adopt this technology. However, perceived ease of use and perceived usefulness may not fully reflect the motivation of users of mobile business applications. Depending on the specific technology context, additional explanatory variables may be needed beyond perceived ease of use and perceived usefulness. Researchers have extended TAM with some additional constructs into the context of e-business and mobile business [15–17]. For example, perceived risk has proved to be an important factor to impact the adoption of E-business [18]. Gao and Krogstie [19] and Gao et al. [20] argued that there were also other non-technical factors that impact users' adoption of mobile services. For entertainment-oriented services, both utilitarian and hedonic aspects are important [21, 22].

## 2.4  The Use of Mobile Business Supporting Features

It is believed that people who get fully use of mobile business supporting features have opportunities to get economic gains offered by mobile business. Therefore, it is important for users to take advantage of the supporting features offered by mobile business applications. The supporting features can be associated with buyers' buying decision-making model. Buying decision-making model has divided the purchasing process into the following five steps [23]: problems cognitive, information search, alternative evaluation, purchase decision and post purchase behavior. Among the five steps, the information search and purchase decision were thought to be the most important steps [24]. Mobile business supporting features is of help for users to make a right buying decision. The objective of this study is to investigate the use of mobile business supporting features with individual with different socio-economic status in China. Compared to E-business applications, mobile business applications have potential to provide more advanced supporting features (e.g., location based services [25]). For example, users can use taxi-hailing application to locate and hail the closet taxi. Concerning the stages involved in buying decision-making model, we focus on studying the use of mobile business supporting features in the information search stage of the purchasing process.

# 3 Research Model and Hypotheses

## 3.1 Research Model

To address the research objective, we built a model to explain how and to what extent socio-economic status influence the use of mobile business supporting features. On the one hand, we applied an expanded TAM model to fit the context of the use of mobile business supporting features. The utilitarian motivations were used to replace perceived usefulness in TAM. Furthermore, the perceived risk and hedonic motivations were added to the original TAM model. The four dependent variables in this research are perceived ease of use, perceived risk, hedonic motivations and utilitarian motivations. The definitions of these four variables are illustrated in Table 1. One the other hand, the socio-economic status was included to the research model as a moderator variable. The research model is presented in Fig. 1.

**Table 1** Construct definitions and sources

| Construct | Definition | Sources |
|---|---|---|
| Perceived ease of use | The degree to which an individual believes that using mobile business supporting features would be free of effort | [14] |
| Perceived risk | The user's subjective expectation of suffering a loss in pursuit of the desired outcome of using mobile business supporting features | [17, 18] |
| Hedonic motivations | The pleasure and inherent satisfaction derived from using mobile business supporting features | [26, 27] |
| Utilitarian motivations | The extent to which using mobile business supporting features enhances the effectiveness of personal related activity | [26, 27] |

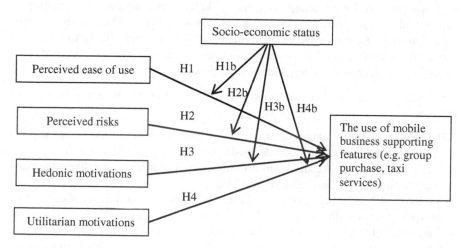

**Fig. 1** Research Model

## 3.2 Research Hypotheses

Borrowed from TAM [14], perceived ease of use reflects how difficult it will be to use a new technology or system. This belief is associated with an individual's assessment of the mental effort involved in using a new technology or system. Mobile services are provided on mobile devices. The limitations of mobile devices may have the potential to affect users' perceptions of ease of use of mobile services. Previous studies (e.g., [16, 28]) have demonstrated that Perceived Ease of Use has a direct positive impact on intention to use mobile services.

Due to the complexity of mobile business supporting features, socio-economically disadvantaged individuals are different to socio-economically advantaged individuals in their perceived ease of use. Socio-economically disadvantaged individuals are usually less effectively than socio-economically advantaged individuals in coping with issues in the process of using mobile technologies. Consequently, the perceived ease of use may have a more intense influence on the use of mobile business supporting features for socio-economically disadvantaged individuals. Therefore, we proposed the hypotheses as follows:

**H1** Perceived ease of use have positive effect on the use of mobile business supporting features.

**H1b** Socio-economic status will moderate the positive relationship between perceived ease of use and the use of mobile business supporting features such that the relationship is stronger for the socio-economically disadvantaged individuals than the socio-economically advantaged individuals.

Perceived risk (PR) is commonly thought of as felt uncertainty regarding possible negative consequences of using a product or service [29]. It is believed that perceived risk would have a negative influence on the use of mobile business supporting features. People with higher income were more likely to take risks [30], while people with lower income were more likely to have an intensive emotional vulnerability with respect to financial losses [31]. Consequently, the socio-economically disadvantaged individuals tend to be more likely to be influenced by perceived risks than the socio-economically advantaged individuals. Therefore, we proposed the hypotheses as follows:

**H2** Perceived risks have a negative effect on the use of mobile business supporting features.

**H2b** Socio-economic status will moderate the positive relationship between perceived risks and the use of mobile business supporting features such that the relationship is stronger for the socio-economically disadvantaged individuals than the socio-economically advantaged individuals.

Hedonic and utilitarian motivations have been proved to have effect on consumer behavior of online shopping [26]. For example, Gao et al. [1] found that utilitarian benefits and perceived enjoyment had a significant positive impact on older adults' intention to use smartphones in China. It is believed that both hedonic motivations and utilitarian motivations would have a positive impact on the use of mobile business supporting features.

Pervious research also revealed that getting utilitarian benefits were more important to the socio-economically advantaged individuals than the socio-economically disadvantaged individuals. For example, Norris [32] suggested that socio-economically advantaged individuals have better opportunities to access and use information technology than socio-economically disadvantaged individuals because of their better level of education. Furthermore, hedonic benefits offered by mobile business applications are more important for the socio-economically disadvantaged individuals than the socio-economically advantaged individuals. The socio-economically disadvantaged individuals were more likely to burden pressures [33]. Using mobile business supporting features is more likely to be seen as a way of stress relief, which is a kind of hedonic motivational drivers, for the socio-economically disadvantaged individuals. Further, socio-economically disadvantaged individuals tend to use mobile services more for entertainment purposes, while socio-economically advantaged individuals tend to use mobile services to facilitate their daily lives. Since socio-economically advantaged individuals are better educated, they are likely to have more experience with mobile services. Thus, they are in a better position to appreciate the usage of mobile business supporting features. Therefore, we proposed the following hypotheses:

**H3** Hedonic motivations have a positive effect on the use of mobile business supporting features.

**H3b** Socio-economic status will moderate the positive relationship between hedonic motivations and the use of mobile business supporting features such that the relationship is stronger for the socio-economically disadvantaged individuals than the socio-economically advantaged individuals.

**H4** Utilitarian motivations have a positive effect on the use of mobile business supporting features.

**H4b** Socio-economic status will moderate the positive relationship between utilitarian motivations and the use of mobile business supporting features such that the relationship is stronger for the socio-economically advantaged individuals than the socio-economically disadvantaged individuals.

# 4 Empirical Study

## 4.1 Instrument Development

Validated instrument measures from previous studies were used as the foundation to create the instrument for this study. In order to ensure that the instrument better fit the context of mobile business supporting features, some minor changes in wording were made to ensure easy interpretation and comprehension of the questions. As a result, 15 measurement items (see Appendix 1) were included in the instrument. A 7-point Likert scale, with 1 being the negative end of the scale (strongly disagree) and 7 being the positive end of the scale (strongly agree), was used to examine participants' responses to all items in this part. In addition, data were analyzed using structural equation modeling (SEM). As for the dependent variable, the participants were required to answer the following question: how many times did you use the mobile business supporting features (e.g., price comparisons site) for mobile shopping in the past year? The participants can choose among six categories (0 time, 1–5 times, 6–10 times, 11–15 times, 16–20 times and above 20 times).

## 4.2 Sample

The survey was conducted in China. We distributed the survey as Internet-based questionnaires individually from March 15 to April 22 2015. We used a paid service from a Chinese research institutions' website to collect the data. A total of 300 responses were collected, while 258 of them were valid. The survey had a response rate of 86 %. The demographic information of the respondents is summarized in Table 2.

## 4.3 Descriptive Results

Some interesting findings from the descriptive analysis are summarized here. Firstly, we noticed that the first item of perceived ease of use "My interaction with the mobile business supporting features is clear and understandable" has the lowest mean value but the highest standard deviation. This implies that the mobile business supporting features needs to be better designed to fit users' needs. Furthermore, the results indicated that the mean value of the hedonic motivation and utilitarian motivations were relatively high (all above 5.1). This means that people have obvious hedonic motivations and utilitarian motivations when they are using the mobile business supporting features. However, this does not necessarily mean that the hedonic motivations and utilitarian motivations have significant positive influence on the use of mobile business supporting features. Further tests on this were presented in the following sections.

## 4.4 Data Analysis

To test the reliability of each construct in the research model, the Internal Consistency of Reliability (ICR) of each construct was tested with Cronbach's Alpha coefficient. As a result, the Cronbach's Alpha values range from 0.883 to 0.904 (see Table 3).

**Table 2** Demographic information of the respondents

| | | Number | Percent (%) |
|---|---|---|---|
| Gender | Male | 122 | 47.29 |
| | Female | 136 | 52.71 |
| Age | Under 18 | 3 | 1.16 |
| | 18–25 | 104 | 40.31 |
| | 26–30 | 77 | 29.84 |
| | 31–40 | 57 | 22.09 |
| | Above 40 | 17 | 6.59 |
| Educated level | Lower-secondary school | 7 | 2.71 |
| | Upper-secondary school | 13 | 5.04 |
| | Undergraduate students | 188 | 72.87 |
| | Master students | 35 | 13.57 |
| | Doctoral students | 2 | 0.78 |
| | Vocational school students | 13 | 5.04 |
| Monthly disposable income | Under 1000 RMB | 30 | 11.63 |
| | 1000–1999 RMB | 38 | 14.73 |
| | 2000–2999 RMB | 53 | 20.54 |
| | 3000–5999 RMB | 89 | 34.50 |
| | 6000–10,000 RMB | 37 | 14.34 |
| | More than 10,000 RMB | 11 | 4.26 |
| Familiarity mobile phone | Very familiar | 108 | 41.86 |
| | Familiar | 122 | 47.29 |
| | Normal | 28 | 10.85 |
| | Not familiar | 0 | 0.00 |

A score of 0.7 is marked as an acceptable reliability coefficient for Cronbach's Alpha [34]. All the constructs were above 0.70. Therefore, the reliability of the scales was quite good.

All measurement items were from the validated items previous research in this study. Furthermore, we used principal component analysis to extract factors. The factor with characteristic root larger than 1 was extracted and the accumulated variance contribution rate was 69.021 %. The standardized loadings were all above 0.5. Therefore, the validity of the scales was good.

The fit of the hypothesized model can be assessed using six commonly used fit indices [35]: Chi-square, Chi-square/df, Normed Fit Index (NFI), Comparative Fit

**Table 3** Reliability statistics

| Scale | Cronbach's alpha | No of items |
|---|---|---|
| Perceived ease of use | 0.890 | 4 |
| Hedonic motivations | 0.883 | 3 |
| Utilitarian motivations | 0.904 | 4 |
| Perceived risks | 0.896 | 4 |

Index (CFI), Root Mean Square Residual (RMR) and Root Mean Square Error of Approximation (RMSEA). CFI was the primary fit-statistic of the six for the purposes of this study, as recommended by [36]. A CFI above 0.90 is indicative of a well-fitting model. According to our result, CFI is above 0.90 in this study. This means that the resulting measurement model has good model-to-data fit.

## 4.5 Results

### 4.5.1 Test of Main Effects

Table 4 presents regression weights. And the results of the structural model main effect were showed in Fig. 2. Perceived ease of use has been proved to have significant positive effect on the use of mobile business supporting features ($P < 0.01$), with a path coefficient of 0.42. Perceived risks have significant negative effect on the use of mobile business supporting features ($P < 0.05$), with a path coefficient of −0.16. Hedonic motivations and Utilitarian motivations have not been found to have a significant positive influence on the use of mobile business supporting features. Thus, H1 and H2 were supported, while H3 and H4 were not supported (showed as dotted lines in Fig. 2) in this study.

**Table 4** Regression weights: (default model)

|  | Estimate | S.E. | C.R. | $P$ |
|---|---|---|---|---|
| Use <— Perceived ease of use | 0.662 | 0.222 | 2.986 | 0.003 |
| Use <— Hedonic motivations | −0.073 | 0.234 | −0.310 | 0.757 |
| Use <— Utilitarian motivations | 0.159 | 0.283 | 0.562 | 0.547 |
| Use <— Perceived risks | −0.256 | 0.118 | −2.170 | 0.030 |

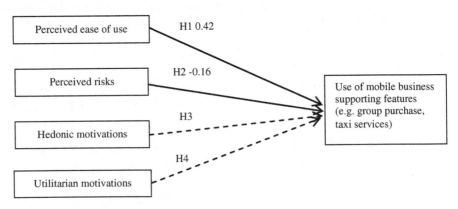

**Fig. 2** Results of structural modeling main effects

### 4.5.2   Tests of Moderating Effects of Socio-Economic Status

Multiple-group analysis in Amos was used to test the moderating effect of socio-economic status. A default model and a limited model have been set up. In the limited model, regression coefficients of perceived ease of use to use of mobile business supporting features between the two groups was set up as equal. The default model was assumed to be correct. The change of chi square value has not been significant at the level $P > 0.05$. Therefore, the results indicated that the socio-economic status did not have a moderating effect on the relationship between perceived ease of use and the use of mobile business supporting features. H1b was not supported. By following the similar approach, we tested the H2b, H3b and H4b. As a result, H2b and H4b were supported, while H3b was not supported. This means that socio-economic status would moderate the relationship between utilitarian motivations and the use of mobile business supporting features such that the relationship is stronger for the socio-economically advantaged individuals than the socio-economically disadvantaged individuals. Furthermore, the results also revealed that socio-economic status would moderate the positive relationship between perceived risks and the use of mobile business supporting features such that the relationship is stronger for the socio-economically disadvantaged individuals than the socio-economically advantaged individuals.

## 5   Discussion

According to the test results, four of eight research hypotheses were supported. Contrary to our expectations, both hedonic motivations and utilitarian motivations did not have significant positive effects on the use of mobile business supporting features. For the hedonic motivations, the possible explanation might be that the mobile business supporting features were not seen as a way to have fun by Chinese consumers. Concerning the utilitarian motivations, some users might not know the possible value of the mobile business supporting features. Moreover, perceived risks had a significant negative effect on the use of mobile business supporting features. This is in consistent with the finding from the previous study that perceived risks was one of the important factors to negatively affect the use of e-business applications [18].

Concerning the moderating effect of socio-economic status, the finding indicated that the relationship between utilitarian motivations and the use of mobile business supporting features was stronger for the socio-economically advantaged individuals than the socio-economically disadvantaged individuals. In the other words, the socio-economically advantaged individuals were more likely to be influenced by the utilitarian motivations. On the other hand, socio-economic status also moderated the relationship between perceived risks and the use of mobile business supporting features. The socio-economically disadvantage individuals were more likely to be influenced by the perceived risks, which confirmed the previous research findings [31].

# 6 Implications

As for the theoretical implications, this study extended the research on digital inequality from the context of E-business to the context of mobile business. This research contributes to the current literature on the use of mobile business supporting features from the perspective of second-order digital inequality. Moreover, the socio-economic status was included into the research model as a moderator. The findings revealed that the socio-economically disadvantage individuals were more likely to be influenced by the perceived risks. However, the socio-economically advantage individuals were more likely to be influenced by the utilitarian motivations.

The mobile devices provided a new channel for users to access the Internet and various applications. Mobile business applications are able to offer potential benefits to consumers. However, these benefits are not equal to all the users. This research also provided some managerial implications to the governmental sector and service providers. For the governmental sector, the results indicated that second-order digital inequality has become a social issue. They need to pay more attention to how mobile business supporting features are used by users. We found that some Internet literacy trainings were needed for the socio-economically disadvantaged individuals to decrease the perceived risks when using mobile business supporting features. Mobile services providers can attempt to attract more users by allowing users to use a trial version of the mobile services without registering their profiles. Having a reliable third party mobile payment service provider can reduce users' perceived risks of mobile business supporting features.

# 7 Conclusion

This study examined the issue of digital inequality in the use of mobile business supporting features in China. A research model with eight research hypotheses was proposed. An empirical study with 258 users was carried out in China. Four research hypotheses were positively significant supported in this research. The results indicated that perceived ease of use had a significant positive effect on the use of mobile business supporting features, while perceived risk had a significant negative effect on the use of mobile business supporting features. Furthermore, this study revealed that socio-economically disadvantaged individuals were more likely to be influenced by perceived risks, while socio-economically advantaged individuals were more likely to be influenced by the utilitarian motivations.

There were also some limitations in this research. First, income and the level of education are just two basic dimensions to define users' socio-economic status. Additional dimension may include in the future research on digital inequality. Second, besides the factors in our structural model, there may have other factors affecting peoples' use of mobile business supporting features. Third, over 70 % of the respondents have an undergraduate degree. This means that most respondents are well educated. This may raises some questions for the findings of this study. Last but not least, the sample size is quite small in this study. The sample may not represent the entire population in China.

## Appendix 1. Survey Instrument

| Factor | Item | Literature |
|---|---|---|
| Perceived ease of use | 1. My interaction with the mobile business supporting features is clear and understandable<br>2. Interacting with the mobile business supporting features do not require a lot of my mental effort<br>3. I find the mobile business supporting features easy to use<br>4. I find it easy to get the mobile business supporting features to do what I want it to do | [27] |
| Hedonic motivations | 1. Using the mobile business supporting features is enjoyable<br>2. Using the mobile business supporting features is pleasant<br>3. Using the mobile business supporting features is fun | [27] |
| Utilitarian motivations | 1. Using the mobile business supporting features improves my performance for information search in the consumption process<br>2. Using the mobile business supporting features improves my productivity for information search in the consumption process<br>3. Using the mobile business supporting features enhances my effectiveness for information search in the consumption process<br>4. Using the mobile business supporting features is useful for my information search in the consumption process | [27] |
| Perceived risk | 1. I think using mobile business supporting features in monetary transactions has potential risk<br>2. I think using mobile business supporting features in product purchase has potential risk<br>3. I think using mobile business supporting features in merchandise services has potential risk<br>4. I think using mobile business supporting features puts my privacy at risk | [17] |

# References

1. Gao, S., Yang, Y., Krogstie, J.: The adoption of smartphones among older adults in china In: Liu, K., Nakata, K., Li, W., et al. (eds.) Information and Knowledge Management in Complex Systems. 449. Springer, Berlin (2015)
2. Buhtz, K., Reinartz, A., König, A., et al.: Second-order digital inequality: the case of e-commerce (2014)
3. DiMaggio, P., Hargittai, E., Celeste, C., et al.: Digital inequality. Social inequality: from unequal access to differentiated use, pp. 355–400 (2004)
4. DiMaggio, P., Hargittai, E.: From the 'digital divide' to 'digital inequality': studying internet use as penetration increases. Princeton: Center for Arts and Cultural Policy Studies, Woodrow Wilson School, Princeton University, vol. 4, no. 1, pp. 4–2 (2001)
5. Katz, J.E., Rice, R.E.: Social consequences of internet use: access, involvement, and interaction. MIT press Cambridge, Cambridge (2002)
6. Hargittai, E.: Second-level digital divide: mapping differences in people's online skills. arXiv preprint cs/0109068 (2001)
7. Mossberger, K., Mary, K.M.C.J.T., Tolbert, C.J., et al.: Virtual inequality: beyond the digital divide. Georgetown University Press, Washington, D.C. (2003)
8. Hargittai, E.: Digital na (t) ives? Variation in internet skills and uses among members of the "net generation". Sociol. Inq. **80**(1), 92–113 (2010)
9. Helbig, N., Gil-García, J.R., Ferro, E.: Understanding the complexity of electronic government: implications from the digital divide literature. Gov. Inf. Q. **26**(1), 89–97 (2009)
10. Chaudhuri, A., Flamm, K.S., Horrigan, J.: An analysis of the determinants of internet access. Telecommun. Policy **29**(9), 731–755 (2005)
11. Rice, R.E., Katz, J.E.: Comparing internet and mobile phone usage: digital divides of usage, adoption, and dropouts. Telecommun. Policy **27**(8), 597–623 (2003)
12. Jung, J.-Y., Qiu, J.L., Kim, Y.-C.: Internet connectedness and inequality beyond the "divide". Commun. Res. **28**(4), 507–535 (2001)
13. Van Deursen, A., Van Dijk, J.: Internet skills and the digital divide. New Media Soc. **13**(6), 893–911 (2011)
14. Davis, F.D.: Perceived usefulness, perceived ease of use and user acceptance of information technology. MIS Q. **13**(3), 319–340 (1989)
15. Gao, S., Krogstie, J., Siau, K.: Developing an instrument to measure the adoption of mobile services. Mobile Inf. Syst. **7**(1), 45–67 (2011)
16. Gao, S., Krogstie, J., Siau, K.: Adoption of mobile information services: an empirical study. Mobile Inf. Syst. **10**(2), 147–171 (2014)
17. Wu, J.-H., Wang, S.-C.: What drives mobile commerce? An empirical evaluation of the revised technology acceptance model. Inf. Manage. **42**(5), 719–729 (2005)
18. Pavlou, P.A.: Consumer acceptance of electronic commerce: integrating trust and risk with the technology acceptance model. Int. J. Electron. Commerce. **7**(3), 101–134 (2003)
19. Gao, S., Krogstie, J.: Explaining the adoption of mobile information services from a cultural perspective. In: The Tenth International Conference on Mobile Business. (ICMB) (2011)
20. Gao, S., Zang, Z., Krogstie, J.: The adoption of mobile games in China: an empirical study. In: Liu, K., Gulliver, S., Li, W., et al. (eds.) Service Science and Knowledge Innovation. 426, 368–377. Springer, Berlin (2014)
21. Gao, S., Krogstie, J., Chen, Z., et al.: Lifestyles and mobile services adoption in China. Int. J. E-Bus. Res. (IJEBR). **10**(3), 36–53 (2014)
22. Haugstvedt, A.-C. and Krogstie, J.: Mobile augmented reality for cultural heritage: a technology acceptance study. pp. 247–255 (2012)
23. Engel, J.F., Kollat, D.T., Blackwell, R.D.: Consumer behavior. New York: holt, rinehart and winston. Inc. Engel2 Consumer Behavior (1973)
24. Gefen, D., Straub, D.W.: The relative importance of perceived ease of use in is adoption: a study of e-commerce adoption. J. Assoc. Inf. Syst. **1**(1), 8 (2000)

25. Gao, S., Krogstie, J., Thingstad, T., et al.: A mobile service using anonymous location-based data: finding reading rooms. Int. J. Inf. Learn. Technol. **32**(1), 32–44 (2015)
26. Childers, T.L., Carr, C.L., Peck, J., et al.: Hedonic and utilitarian motivations for online retail shopping behavior. J. Retail. **77**(4), 511–535 (2002)
27. Hsieh, J.P.-A., Rai, A., Keil, M.: Understanding digital inequality: comparing continued use behavioral models of the socio-economically advantaged and disadvantaged. MIS Q. 97–126 (2008)
28. Gao, S., Moe, S.P., Krogstie, J.: An empirical test of the mobile services acceptance model. In: The Proceedings of the 9th International Conference on Mobile Business and the Ninth Global Mobility Roundtable (ICMB-GMR 2010), pp. 168–175 (2010)
29. Featherman, M.S., Pavlou, P.A.: Predicting e-services adoption: a perceived risk facets perspective. Int. J. Hum Comput Stud. **59**(4), 451–474 (2003)
30. Schechter, L.: Risk aversion and expected-utility theory: a calibration exercise. J. Risk Uncertainty **35**(1), 67–76 (2007)
31. McLeod, J.D., Kessler, R.C.: Socioeconomic status differences in vulnerability to undesirable life events. J. Health Soc. Behav. 162–172 (1990)
32. Norris, P.: Digital divide: civic engagement, information poverty, and the internet worldwide. Cambridge University Press, Cambridge (2001)
33. Aneshensel, C.S.: Social stress: theory and research. Ann. Rev. Sociol. 15–38 (1992)
34. Kline, P.: The handbook of psychological testing. Routledge, London (1993)
35. Iacobucci, D.: Structural equations modeling: fit indices, sample size, and advanced topics. J. Consum. Psychol. **20**(1), 90–98 (2010)
36. Bentler, P.M.: On the fit of models to covariances and methodology to the bulletin. Psychol. Bull. **112**(3), 400 (1992)

# Understanding Problematic Smartphone Use and Its Characteristics: A Perspective on Behavioral Addiction

Chuang Wang, Matthew K.O. Lee, Chen Yang and Xiaodong Li

**Abstract** The problematic use of smartphones has drawn increasing attention because of harmful and disturbing outcomes. However, there has been little comprehensive research concerning the mechanism of problematic behavior in the use of smartphones, particularly for behavioral addiction. Given the specific characteristics of smartphones (e.g., high mobility, instant connection, and ubiquitous access), it is highlighted that smartphone addiction is a behavior that differs from traditional addiction behavior. However, in previous research, there is a lack of comprehensive understanding of the characteristics and the underlying mechanisms of smartphone addiction. Motivated to systematically theorize this issue, we primarily define addiction in the smartphone context and comprehend the characteristics of smartphone addiction, followed by developing the measures for smartphone addiction. On this conceptual foundation, future empirical research should be able to explain, predict, and test addiction behavior in the use of smartphones.

**Keywords** Problematic smartphone use · Addiction behavior · Smartphone

A prior version of this paper has been published in the ISD2015 Proceedings (http://aisel.aisnet.org/isd2014/proceedings2015/).

C. Wang (✉)
South China University of Technology, Guangzhou, China
e-mail: bmchwang@scut.edu.cn; lincywang1988@gmail.com

M.K.O. Lee
City University of Hong Kong, Hong Kong, China
e-mail: matthew.k.o.lee@cityu.edu.hk

C. Yang
Shenzhen University, Shenzhen, China
e-mail: yangc0201@gmail.com

X. Li
University of Science and Technology of China, Hefei, China
e-mail: lxd512@mail.ustc.edu.cn

© Springer International Publishing Switzerland 2016
D. Vogel et al. (eds.), *Transforming Healthcare Through Information Systems*,
Lecture Notes in Information Systems and Organisation 17,
DOI 10.1007/978-3-319-30133-4_15

# 1  Introduction

Smartphones and other mobile computing devices have become a daily part of our lives. With the great improvement of electronic technology and the rapid influx of new applications introduced to the public, smartphones can serve various functions such as providing instant news, web browsing, text messaging, online gaming, online shopping, social networking, and so forth. Nowadays people use smartphones very frequently—smartphones have become the first things many of us reach for when we wake up in the morning and frequently the last thing we check before going to sleep at night [1]. For the majority of individuals, smartphones represent an incredible tool for information update, instant communication, social connection, self-education, and entertainment. The use of mobile devices is a normal and routine part of everyday life. However, for some users, they look at their phones' menu screens, news, emails and apps throughout the day. The failure to control an overwhelming impulse to check their phones pervades their lives and results in negative consequences.

As our dependency on mobile technology grows, an increasing attention has been paid to the use of smartphones. Particularly, we found a significant number of studies on negative consequences of mobile phone use. Most of these studies dealt with ill-effects or ill-coordination of mobile phones use. For example, researchers examined the possible adverse health issues of mobile phones [2–4] and phone-related driving hazards [5–7]. In recent years, there are an increasing number of studies on negative psychological effects on the smartphone usage, particularly from psychiatrists, psychologists, and social psychologists. However, existing studies tend to adopt a traditional and general way as an exploration of problematic smartphone use in nature. For instance, most studies focused on demographics and personality traits of mobile phone users [8–10], as well as dimensions and measurement instruments of problematic smartphone use [11, 12]. Some researchers addressed diagnoses, symptom management and treatment strategies for addictive mobile phone use [13, 14].

Theory-guided studies on the development of addictive smartphone use are relatively rare. There is little understanding of the process of addiction IS/IT behavior, as well as the variables affecting its enactment. The scant theoretical research might be attributed to a lack of a common nomenclature and conceptualization, which is crucial in providing the conceptual foundation and developing a useful theory [15, 16]. Therefore, this study aims at enriching existing IS literature on addictive use of technologies by primarily developing the conceptual foundation for addiction behavior in the context of smartphones and identifying its specific characteristics.

Important theoretical and practical contributions are expected from this study. On the theoretical side, this research project addressing addictive use of technologies will enrich existing IS literature by augmenting our knowledge of typical system usage. Particularly, our result will illustrate how the key characteristics of addictive use operate to drive addictive smartphone use. On the practical side, this investigation is timely to enhance our understanding of the problematic usage of smartphones, a seemingly universal phenomenon. The results will help clinicians, educators, and parents to develop possible counter-measures against addictive use of smartphones.

## 2 Theoretical Background

### 2.1 Prior Literature

Though research on problematic use of IS/IT is still evolving in the IS field, a significant number of studies on smartphone-related addiction have been conducted in the psychology and clinical psychology literature [17, 18]. For instance, Kwon et al. [19] proposed a series of scales to identify the addiction symptoms of smartphone use, measuring as daily-life disturbance, positive anticipation, withdrawal, cyberspace-oriented relationship, overuse, and tolerance. Similarly, Casey [11] defined smartphone addiction as a set of symptoms such as disregard of harmful consequences, preoccupation, inability to control craving, productivity loss, and feeling anxious and lost. However, scholars have been limited by a lack of deep understanding in this area. Our review of prior studies found that previous studies mainly focused on demographics and psychosocial characteristics of mobile phone users [17, 20], and dimensions and measurement instruments [11, 21].

Based on the critical review mentioned above, research in the field of "problematic use of smartphone" is still explorative and evolving. There has been no consensus on the causes and consequences, and even no consensus has been reached on the nomenclature used to describe the phenomenon. In the previous literature concerning about the smartphone use, this type of irrational behavior has been referred as addiction [11, 12, 19, 21–24], compulsive usage [20, 25], and problematic use [17]. In this article, we prefer the term addiction because it represents a behavioral pattern that causes compulsive use despite harmful consequences [26]. A review of prior literature found that addiction behaviors occur in various technology use, such as online gaming, social network, instant messaging, online gambling and so forth, and they share a number of common features. These include psychological dependence, loss of control, and negative consequences related to everyday life [27, 28].

## 2.2 Characteristics of Smartphone Addiction

Although addiction behavior has been pervasively investigated in prior literature, it has been highlighted that "studies are still needed to explore the similarities and differences between smartphone addiction and other behavioral addictions" [17, p. 303]. Similarly, it is proposed that understanding the characteristics of mobile addiction is useful and effective in capturing the usage behavior and motivation of smartphone use [29]. Following this line of reasoning, we primarily identify the characteristics of smartphone addiction (as shown in Table 1). We further proposed the underlying mechanism of such characteristics as an integration of rewarding base with compensation base, discussed in the following paragraphs.

## 2.3 Conceptualization of Smartphone Addiction

Typically, IT addiction has been defined as "the dependency to a technology that results in its excessive and compulsive use" [33, p. 1064]. Consistent with this

**Table 1** Characteristics of smartphone addiction

| Characteristics | Description | Underlying mechanisms |
|---|---|---|
| Ubiquitous | "Habits make smartphone use more pervasive" [30] | Rewarding base |
| Socially accepted, normal | "The guise of a 'normal' socially acceptable activity" [31] | |
| Natural, undetectable, habit-forming | A checking habit [30]; A natural part of today's life, check smartphone over and over without even thinking about it [32] | |
| Voluntary | A reasoned behavior for social and personal benefits on the basis of positive attitudes and social norms [29]; "A desired behavior that can facilitate tasks and help improving performance" [33]; Positive experiences of repetitive uses [30] | |
| Mandatory | Using smartphones is necessary to daily lives [20], [29] The feelings of missing out [25] Anxiety and withdrawal [34] | Compensation base |
| Session usage | More shorter non-even-initiated interaction sessions (i.e., the interval between the screen turning on and the screen turning off) evenly spread over the day [35]; Short, brief usage sessions repeating over time [30] | |
| Contextual, stimulus-oriented | Tightly associated with a particular triggering context (e.g., bus trip, lecture, and home) [30, 36]; Driven or prompted by environmental consequences [20, 29] | |
| Annoyance, rather than conflict | Not yet perceived as problematic [30] | |

definition, Thadani and Cheung [37] proposed that addiction acts as the compulsive repetition elicited by psychological dependence. From this perspective, addiction is perceived as a type of irrational behaviour that results in negative consequences on individuals.

By identifying the characteristics of smartphone addiction, we attempt to explain the rationale of smartphone addiction through differentiating it from traditional addiction behavior. First, smartphone addiction is conducted as a reinforcement process associated with desired rewarding experience [38]. Given that smartphones allow users to pursue their instant connection anytime and anywhere [20, 36], the high responsiveness of smartphone is of great value for individuals [39]. In this case, repetitive usage pattern for the gratification of interactivity and connectivity (i.e., the rewarding experience) is readily developed. From this perspective, smartphone addiction is perceived as a normal, socially accepted, and seemingly harmless habit, performing voluntarily in the pursuit of rewarding experience.

Second, smartphone addiction is also performed to compensate the none-use experience of smartphone usage. Compulsion occurs with "a chronic, repetitive, and excessive behavioral response to inner deficiencies, negative feelings and events" [40, p. 510]. Given the feelings of missing out [25], anxiety and withdrawal [34], individuals defensively approach the smartphone usage to overcome the potential threatens of none-use, thus leading to smartphone addiction as a necessary and mandatory part in daily life. In summary, we propose that smartphone addiction as users' repetitive and persistent checking behavior with the goal to maximize potential rewarding experience and compensate potential threatens.

# 3  Research Methodology

As research on addictive use of IS/IT is evolving, the conceptualization and operationalization of addiction are still in the development stage [41]. Particularly, the crucial construct (i.e., smartphone addiction) has not been investigated in the context of mobile technologies. Therefore, we focus on the conceptualization of smartphone addiction, and develop measures specific to the context of the current study by following Moore and Benbasat's [42] instrument development approach.

## 3.1  The Inconsistence of Addiction Measurement

Although existing studies have developed a plethora of measures for addiction, no consensus has been reached to date. Despite the considerable merits of previous measurements, we believe that there still exist several limitations on the basis of our conceptualization of smartphone addiction.

First, addiction should be distinguished from similar constructs, such as compulsion, dependence, and problematic use. Studies that investigate the inappropriate use of smartphone typically adopt a set of nomenclature, while departing the definition of the construct from its measurement. A confusion of the research unit may lead to the failure to understand its underlying mechanisms. Therefore, a fine-grained threshold for smartphone addiction should be proposed, albeit the difference of these constructs is significantly subtle.

Second, addiction should be defined with a difference from its antecedents and consequences. The overlaps of addiction with its antecedents (e.g., mood modification, positive anticipation) and consequences (e.g., conflict, disturbance) have been pervasively found in previous addiction research [19, 41]. Despite the high relatedness of these factors to addiction, it is believed that they cannot be conceived as the addiction behavior in nature.

Finally, addiction should be measured with a focus on the behavior itself, rather than the interplay of emotional and cognitional process. It has been highlighted that the essence of addiction is an uncontrolled behavior to repetitively engage in the specific behaviour [17]. Well in line with this perspective, Griffiths [43, p. 211] proposed that "technological addiction acts as a behavioral addiction that involves human-technology interaction, rather than a chemical addiction". From this perspective, addiction should be distinguished from the emotion or belief systems. Given the inconsistencies of addiction measurement, we believe that it is imperative to develop a proper measurement for addiction in the context of smartphone use.

## 3.2   Measurement for Smartphone Addiction

To refine the conceptualization and operationalization of smartphone addiction, we start the measurement based on the assumptions in the following.

We first assume that smartphone addiction is different from online auction, gambling, and gaming addiction. Rather, it acts as a behavioral pattern of individuals' uncontrollable urges to repetitively check their smartphones. Given that smartphones provide a seminal platform for information obtainment and social connection, individuals are spurred to consecutively use their smartphones to pursue those neutral and even positive aspects of smartphones. Technological attributes of smartphones such as interactivity and mobility lead to the proportion of smartphone addiction far greater than any other known so far. In this regard, the criteria such that "addiction occurs depending on its negative impacts on society, family, and individuals themselves" might be not suitable in the mobile context. Instead, smartphone addiction tends to be more pervasive and social facilitating in comparison with other problematic technology use. Following this line of reasoning, we believe that it is not necessary to clarify the significant difference between addicts and non-addicts. Oppositely, each user is conceived as a potential of addict, albeit with a varying extent.

We then define smartphone addiction as a reflective construct, with the focus on behavioral addiction. Contrasted with previous studies that define addiction as a multiple-dimension construct [11, 12, 21], we believe a concise definition that focuses on the addiction behavior itself, rather than the containing of its antecedents and consequences, is more appropriate to provide the fundamental theoretical base of smartphone addiction.

Finally, we clarify smartphone addiction as a behavioral salience. This is mainly because that "salience" (i.e., preoccupation) is the fundamental base of addiction. IT addictive behaviors have been defined as "IT-related behaviors that become a major focus of a person's life and that have potential negative consequences" [33, p. 1064]. Consistent with this definition, evidence from the previous studies has been demonstrated that the majority symptoms such as withdrawal, conflict, relapse, tolerance, and mood modification simultaneously occur with salience [41]. Moreover, "the excessive levels of use, craving, structuring other activities around the addiction behavior, or feeling arousal while using" can be well represented by "preoccupation" [44]—a symptom that can be interchangeably described as salience. Therefore, we conceptualize smartphone addiction as a set of behaviors that saliently dominate individuals' daily life.

Based on these assumptions, we initially reviewed a great deal of literature on smartphone addiction, compulsion, and dependence, and rule out those measures that distract addiction behavior from symptoms such as "withdrawal", "mood modification", and "relapse and reinstatement". We then provide a basic operationalization of smartphone addiction on the basis of previous literature [11, 12, 19, 21, 45]. The items such that "I frequently check my smartphone," "I use my smartphone any time I can," "I often check my smartphone before something else that I need to do," "I often find myself engaged on the smartphone for longer period of time than intended," and "I often find myself anticipating when I will use the smartphone again" pave a seminal venue to measure addiction behavior in the context of smartphone use.

To test the validity of the items for smartphone addiction, we invited 56 active smartphone users to participate in a pilot study to refine the clarity of the questionnaire. Invitations were carried out by posting in various popular smartphone communities in China. To encourage participation, we gave remuneration to each participant. As the pilot study proceeded without any problem, it is evidenced that our measurement development was appropriate, and the questionnaire was understandable and operational. Table 2 describes the details of the results for reliability and validity.

# 4 Discussion and Conclusion

This research seeks to advance the understanding of addictive use of smartphones. Though addiction has been widely studied in psychology, pathology, and biology, there are few systematic theoretical studies that explain and predict the smartphonee

**Table 2** The preliminary results for reliability and validity

| No. | Item | Mean | S.D | Factor loading | Cronbach's α | AVE |
|-----|------|------|-----|----------------|--------------|-----|
| 1 | I frequently check my smartphone | 4.93 | 0.083 | 0.801 | 0.852 | 0.630 |
| 2 | I use my smartphone any time I can | 4.83 | 0.084 | 0.823 | | |
| 3 | I often check my smartphone before something else that I need to do | 4.01 | 0.089 | 0.808 | | |
| 4 | I often find myself engaged on the smartphone for longer period of time than intended | 4.86 | 0.080 | 0.793 | | |
| 5 | I often find myself anticipating when I will use the smartphone again | 3.92 | 0.084 | 0.740 | | |

addiction in IS research. One possible explanation is that the distinct nomenclature and conceptualization lead to a divergent theoretical base for understanding the causal mechanism of addiction behavior.

We identified the characteristics of smartphone addiction to understand and capture the addiction behavior in the use of smartphone. Our conceptualization integrates the rewarding experience with compensative experience, both of which exert a joint effect on the development of smartphone addiction. Based on this finding, we proposed a comprehensive understanding about smartphone addiction, which can be used by researchers and practitioners for further explaining its theoretical foundation.

We also expect this research project to yield important practical contributions. Although the problematic use of smartphone seems as a harmless habit, it has led to a harmful and disturbing outcome to the individuals and the society [17]. Our theoretical investigation is timely and imperative to enhance our understanding about the characteristics and underlying process of smartphone addiction. The expected results will help people to capture, predict, and understand the processes toward the development of addictive use of smartphone.

Aside from the empirical test of our theoretical mechanism, there still exist several factors that draw our attention. First, the technological attributes of smartphone (e.g., mobility, interactivity, pervasive access, and ease of use) facilitate the development of addiction behavior and contribute to the act of urge associated with the repetitive checking. In this regard, the theoretical understanding could be expanded to consider the role of technological attributes in the form of smartphone addiction.

Second, individuals' personality (e.g., low self-esteem, depression) also introduces theoretical possibilities in explaining the addiction behavior. Previous studies have shown that people who have certain personality and social-psychological characteristics are more likely to develop problematic use of technologies [11, 17, 46–48]. Whether the internal personality of individuals plays a role in the development of smartphone addiction needs further empirical research.

**Acknowledgments** The work described in this paper was substantially supported by "the Fundamental Research Funds for the Central Universities" (Project No.2015QNXM10) and China Postdoctoral Science Foundation (Project No. 2015M582389).

# References

1. Perlow, L.A.: Sleeping with Your Smartphone: How to Break the 24/7 Habit and Change the Way You Work. Harvard Business Review Press, Boston (2012)
2. Hocking, B.: Preliminary report: symptoms associated with mobile phone use. Occup. Med. **48**(6), 357–360 (1998)
3. Lönn, S., Ahlbom, A., Hall, P., Feychting, M.: Long-term mobile phone use and brain tumor risk. Am. J. Epidemiol. **161**(6), 526–535 (2005)
4. Lahkola, A., Auvinen, A., Raitanen, J., Schoemaker, M.J., Christensen, H.C., Feychting, M., Swerdlow, A.J.: Mobile phone use and risk of glioma in 5 north European countries. Int. J. Cancer **120**(8), 1769–1775 (2007)
5. Haigney, D., Taylor, R., Westerman, S.: Concurrent mobile (cellular) phone use and driving performance: task demand characteristics and compensatory processes. Trans. Res. Part F: Traffic Psychol. Behav. **3**(3), 113–121 (2000)
6. Hancock, P., Lesch, M., Simmons, L.: The distraction effects of phone use during a crucial driving maneuver. Accid. Anal. Prev. **35**(4), 501–514 (2003)
7. White, M.P., Eiser, J.R., Harris, P.R.: Risk perceptions of mobile phone use while driving. Risk Anal. **24**(2), 323–334 (2004)
8. Billieux, J., Van der Linden, M., d'Acremont, M., Ceschi, G., Zermatten, A.: Does impulsivity relate to perceived dependence on and actual use of the mobile phone? Appl. Cogn. Psychol. **21**(4), 527–537 (2007)
9. James, D., Drennan, J.: Exploring addictive consumption of mobile phone technology. In: The Australian and New Zealand Marketing Academy Conference, pp. 87–96. Perth, Australia (2005)
10. Takao, M., Takahashi, S., Kitamura, M.: Addictive personality and problematic mobile phone use. Cyberpsychology Behav. **12**(5), 501–507 (2009)
11. Casey, B.M.: Linking psychological attributes to smart phone addiction, face-to-face communication, present absence and social capital. Master's Thesis, The Chinese University of Hong Kong (2012)
12. Koo, H.Y.: Development of a cell phone addiction scale for Korean adolescents. J. Korean Acad. Nurs. **39**(6), 818–828 (2009)
13. Beranuy, M., Oberst, U., Carbonell, X., Chamarro, A.: Problematic internet and mobile phone use and clinical symptoms in college students: the role of emotional intelligence. Comput. Hum. Behav. **25**(5), 1182–1187 (2009)
14. Yen, C.-F., Tang, T.-C., Yen, J.-Y., Lin, H.-C., Huang, C.-F., Liu, S.-C., Ko, C.-H.: Symptoms of problematic cellular phone use, functional impairment and its association with depression among adolescents in Southern Taiwan. J. Adolesc. **32**(4), 863–873 (2009)
15. Lowry, P.B., Curtis, A., Lowry, M.R.: Building a taxonomy and nomenclature of collaborative writing to improve interdisciplinary research and practice. J. Bus. Commun. **41**(1), 66–99 (2004)
16. Posey, C., Roberts, T., Lowry, P.B., Bennett, B., Courtney, J.: Insiders' protection of organizational information assets: development of a systematics-based taxonomy and theory of diversity for protection-motivated behaviors. MIS Q. **37**(4), 1189–1210 (2013)
17. Billieux, J.: Problematic use of the mobile phone: a literature review and a pathways model. Curr. Psychiatry Rev. **8**(4), 299–307 (2012)
18. Sarwar, M., Soomro, T.R.: Impact of smartphone's on society. Eur. J. Sci. Res. **98**(2), 216–226 (2013)

19. Kwon, M., Lee, J.-Y., Won, W.-Y., Park, J.-W., Min, J.-A., Hahn, C., Kim, D.-J.: Development and validation of a smartphone addiction scale (SAS). PLoS ONE **8**(2), 1–7 (2013)

20. Park, B.-W., Lee, K.C.: The effect of users' characteristics and experiential factors on the compulsive usage of the smartphone. In: Kim, T.-H., Adeli, H., Robles, R.J., Balitanas, M. (eds.) Ubiquitous Computing and Multimedia Applications—Communications in Computer and Information Science, vol. 151, pp. 438–446. Springer, Berlin (2011)

21. Leung, L.: Unwillingness-to-communicate and college students' motives in sms mobile messaging. Telematics Inform. **24**(2), 115–129 (2007)

22. Roberts, J.A., Pirog, S.F.: A preliminary investigation of materialism and impulsiveness as predictors of technological addictions among young adults. J. Behav. Addict. **2**(1), 56–62 (2013)

23. Salehan, M., Negahban, A.: Social networking on smartphones: when mobile phones become addictive. Comput. Hum. Behav. **29**(6), 2632–2639 (2013)

24. Wu, A.M., Cheung, V.I., Ku, L., Hung, E.P.: Psychological risk factors of addiction to social networking sites among chinese smartphone users. J. Behav. Addict. **2**(3), 160–166 (2013)

25. Hoetjes, M.: (Compulsive) Mobile phone checking behavior out of a fear of missing out: development, psychometric properties and test-retest reliability of a c-fomo-scale (2013)

26. Association psychiatric association: diagnostic criteria from Dsm-Iv-Tr. Amer Psychiatric Publishing Incorporated (2000)

27. Goodman, A.: Addiction: definition and implications. Br. J. Addict. **85**(11), 1403–1408 (1990)

28. Russell, M.: Tobacco dependence: is nicotine rewarding or aversive? In: Krasnegor, N.A. (ed.) Cigarette Smoking as a Dependence Process, pp. 100–122. Government Printing Office, Washington DC (1979)

29. Hooper, V., Zhou, Y.: Addictive, dependent, compulsive? A study of mobile phone usage. In: Proceedings of the 20th Bled eConference e-Mergence: Merging and Emerging Technologies, Processes, and Institutions, pp. 272–285. Slovenia (2007)

30. Oulasvirta, A., Rattenbury, T., Ma, L., Raita, E.: Habits make smartphone use more pervasive. Pers. Ubiquit. Comput. **16**(1), 105–114 (2012)

31. Wright, J.: The Soft Addiction Solution: Break Free of the Seemingly Harmless Habits that Keep you from the Life you Want. Tarcher, New York, NY (2006)

32. Ahn, J., Jung, Y.: The common sense of dependence on smartphone: a comparison between digital natives and digital immigrants. New Media Soc. 15 Oct (2014)

33. Lapointe, L., Boudreau-Pinsonneault, C., Vaghefi, I.: Is smartphone usage truly smart? A qualitative investigation of it addictive behaviors. In: The Proceedings of the 46th Hawaii International Conference on Information Systems, pp. 1063–1072. Wailea, Maui, HI (2013)

34. Sidhaarthaa.: Cisco report: 90 % of gen y compulsively check their smartphones for updates. Acceesed from 15 Jan 2015 http://wirelessduniya.com/2012/12/14/60-of-gen-y-compulsively-check-their-smartphones-for-updates/ (2012)

35. Shin, C., Dey, A.K.: Automatically detecting problematic use of smartphones. In: The Proceedings of the 2013 ACM International Joint Conference on Pervasive and Ubiquitous Computing, pp. 335–344. Zurich, Switerland (2013)

36. Malinen, S., Ojala, J.: Maintaining the instant connection—social media practices of smartphone Users. In: Dugdale, J., Masclet, C., Grasso, M.A., Boujut, J.-F., Hassanaly, P. (eds.) From Research to Practice in the Design of Cooperative Systems: Results and Open Challenges, pp. 197–211. Springer, London (2012)

37. Thadani, D.R., Cheung, C.M.: Online social network dependency: theoretical development and testing of competing models. In: The Proceedings of the 44th Hawaii International Conference on Information Systems, Kauai, HI, pp. 1–9 (2011)

38. Hursh, S.R., Silberberg, A.: Economic demand and essential value. Psychol. Rev. **115**(1), 186–198 (2008)

39. Zhao, L., Lu, Y.: Enhancing perceived interactivity through network externalities: an empirical study on micro-blogging service satisfaction and continuance intention. Decis. Support Syst. **53**(4), 825–834 (2012)

40. Neuner, M., Raab, G., Reisch, L.A.: Compulsive buying in maturing consumer societies: an empirical re-inquiry. J. Econ. Psychol. **26**(4), 509–522 (2005)
41. Turel, O., Serenko, A., Giles, P.: Integrating technology addiction and use: an empirical investigation of online auction users. MIS Q. **35**(4), 1043–1061 (2011)
42. Moore, G.C., Benbasat, I.: Development of an instrument to measure the perceptions of adopting an information technology innovation. Inf. Syst. Res. **2**(3), 192–222 (1991)
43. Griffiths, M.: Does internet and computer "addiction" exist? Some case study evidence. Cyberpsychology Behav. **3**(2), 211–218 (2000)
44. Larose, R., Lin, C.A., Eastin, M.S.: Unregulated internet usage: addiction, habit, or deficient self-regulation? Media Psychol. **5**(3), 225–253 (2003)
45. Young, K.S.: Internet addiction: the emergence of a new clinical disorder. Cyberpsychology Behav. **1**(3), 237–244 (2009)
46. Caplan, S.E.: Problematic internet use and psychosocial well-being: development of a theory-based cognitive-behavioral measurement instrument. Comput. Hum. Behav. **18**(5), 553–575 (2002)
47. Davis, R.A.: A cognitive-behavioral model of pathological internet use. Comput. Hum. Behav. **17**(2), 187–195 (2001)
48. Widyanto, L., Griffiths, M.: 'Internet addiction': a critical review. Int. J. Ment. Health Addict. **4**(1), 31–51 (2006)

Printed in the United States
By Bookmasters